C0-CFV-577

IS SIZE

IMPORTANT?

IS SIZE

IMPORTANT?

by
Donald I. Templer, Ph.D.
California School of Professional Psychology – Fresno

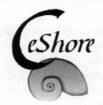

Pittsburgh, PA

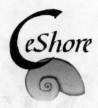

ISBN 1-58501-032-4

Trade Paperback
© Copyright 2002 Donald I. Templer Ph.D.
All rights reserved
First Printing—2002
Library of Congress #2001096828

Request for information should be addressed to:

CeShore
SterlingHouse Publisher, Inc.
7436 Washington Avenue
Suite #200
Pittsburgh, PA 15218
www.sterlinghousepublisher.com

Cover design: Michelle S. Lenkner - SterlingHouse Publisher
Book Designer: N. J. McBeth
CeShore is an imprint of SterlingHouse Publisher, Inc.

The information in this book is not intended to take the place of
medical advice or treatment.

All rights reserved. No part of this publication may be reproduced,
stored in a retrieval system, or transmitted in any form or by any
means—electronic, mechanical, photocopy, recording or any other,
except for brief quotations in printed reviews—without prior
permission of the publisher.

Printed in The United States of America

IS SIZE IMPORTANT?

TABLE OF CONTENTS

PAGE

INTRODUCTION 1

CHAPTER 1 – Penis Growth from Birth
to Adulthood 3

CHAPTER 2 – What is Average? What is
Big? What is Small? 13

CHAPTER 3 – Size of the Penis and the
Size of the Man 37

CHAPTER 4 – Racial Differences in
Penis Size 43

CHAPTER 5 – Abnormally Small Penis Size 57

CHAPTER 6 – What Size Penises Women
Prefer 63

CHAPTER 7 – Penis Size in Fantasies
of Women 95

CHAPTER 8 – Methods Used to Increase
Penis Size 107

CHAPTER 9 – Conclusions 119

WORKS CITED 125

INTRODUCTION

Penis size is what this book is all about. It is about penis size and nothing but penis size. Although much of the material used for this book comes from the medical and scientific literature, it is written in plain language so that the average person can understand.

Who is interested in penis size? Almost all people have at least some interest in penis size. Most people who say they don't are lying. A large percentage of sexual jokes, and even some racial jokes, pertain to penis size; e.g., the man who was arrested for indecent exposure but later released because of insufficient evidence. Men in the locker rooms appraise the penis size of other men while pretending not to even notice that the other men have penises. Men are chosen for pornographic movies on the basis of penis size. In some cultures, size of the penis of a newborn boy is talked about. Many men take pride in being "well hung," and even more men feel inadequate about their penis size.

We will see that some of the "myths" about sex have elements of truth. Black men do tend to have larger penises than white men. Tall men do tend to have larger penises than short men. Many women do obtain greater pleasure from larger penises. On the other hand, there are also many women who obtain greater pleasure from smaller penises. Also, it sometimes happens that a man's penis is too large for a woman's vagina so that she experiences pain.

Is length or thickness of the penis more important? Is my penis large or average or small? How important is the size of a woman's vagina? Should penis size be taken into consideration in choosing sexual positions? Can surgery make my penis larger? What size penises do Asian men have?

This book helps to answer questions you may have had for a long time.

CHAPTER 1

PENIS GROWTH FROM BIRTH TO ADULTHOOD

The research on penis size and growth from birth to adulthood most cited is that of Schonfeld and Beebe (1948). These researchers measured the penis of 1,480 American white males from birth to 23 years of age. They determined both length and circumference in a flaccid, but stretched to full length state. They requested 150 subjects to measure their erect penis at home and to mail the measurements back on a post card. Schonfeld and Beebe found that the stretched penis length measurements were almost identical to the self-measured erect penis length measurements. They therefore felt confident that stretched penis length was an excellent measure of erect length. Table 1.1 displays the average length, 10th percentile, and 90th percentile from infancy to maturity for the Schonfeld and Beebe study. If a male is at the 90th percentile, his stretched penis length is in the upper 10% for males his age. A male at the 10th percentile is in the bottom 10%. Table 1.2 is a comparable table for penis circumference.

Nakamura (1961), with 1,528 Japanese subjects from infancy to adulthood, used the same method as Schonfeld and Beebe (1948). Table 1.3 contains the average length, 16th percentile, and 84th percentile, for Japanese stretched penis length at various ages. Table 1.4 presents the same respective information pertaining to circumference.

Table 1.1 Stretched American average penis length at various ages in Schonfeld and Beebe (1942) study.

Age (years)	Length (inches)		
	10%	Average	90%
0-5 months	1	1 1/2	2
6-11 months		1 5/8	
1		1 3/4	
	1 3/8		2 3/8
2		2	
3		2 1/8	
	1 5/8		2 3/4
4		2 1/4	
5		2 3/8	
	1 7/8		2 7/8
6		2 3/8	
7		2 3/8	
	1 7/8		3
8		2 1/2	
9		2 3/8	
	1 7/8		3
10		2 1/2	
11	1 7/8	2 1/2	4 1/2
12	1 7/8	2 3/4	4 7/8
13	2 3/8	3 1/2	5 3/8
14	2 5/8	3 7/8	5 3/8
15	3 3/8	4 5/8	5 7/8
16	4 1/4	4 7/8	6
17	4 1/4	5 1/4	6
18-19	4 1/4	5 1/8	6 1/8
20-25	4 1/2	5 1/8	6 1/8

It should be noted that for the 10th percentile and 90th percentile the 2 under 1 year categories were combined by Schonfeld and Beebe as were ages 1 & 2, ages 3 & 4, ages 5 & 6, ages 7 & 8, and ages 9 & 10.

Donald I. Templer, Ph.D.

Table 1.2 Stretched American average penis circumference at various ages in Schonfeld and Beebe (1942) study.

Age (years)	Length (inches)		
	10%	Average	90%
0-5 months		1 3/8	
	1 1/4		1 5/8
6-11 months		1 1/2	
1		1 1/2	
	1 3/8		1 3/4
2		1 5/8	
3		1 5/8	
	1 3/8		1 3/4
4		1 5/8	
5		1 5/8	
	1 1/2		1 7/8
6		1 3/4	
7		1 5/8	
	1 1/2		2
8		1 3/4	
9		1 3/4	
	1 1/2		2
10		1 7/8	
11	1 5/8	2	2 1/2
12	1 3/4	2 1/4	3
13	1 3/4	2 3/4	3 1/4
14	1 7/8	3	3 3/8
15	2 3/8	3 1/8	3 5/8
16	2 3/8	3 3/8	3 5/8
17	2 3/4	3 1/4	4
18-19	2 3/4	3 3/8	4
20-25	2 7/8	3 3/8	3 7/8

It should be noted that for the 10th percentile and 90th percentile the 2 under 1 year categories were combined by Schonfeld and Beebe as were ages 1 & 2, ages 3 & 4, ages 5 & 6, ages 7 & 8, and ages 9-10.

Table 1.3 Stretched Japanese penis length at various ages with 1,578 subjects in Nakamura (1964) study.

Age (years)	Length (inches)		
	16%	Average	84%
0	1	1	1 1/8
1	1	1 1/8	1 1/4
2	1 1/8	1 1/4	1 1/2
3	1 1/4	1 3/8	1 1/2
4	1 1/4	1 1/2	1 5/8
5	1 3/8	1 5/8	1 3/4
6	1 3/8	1 5/8	1 3/4
7	1 1/2	1 5/8	1 3/4
8	1 1/2	1 5/8	1 7/8
9	1 1/2	1 5/8	1 7/8
10	1 5/8	1 3/4	2
11	1 3/4	1 7/8	2 1/8
12	1 7/8	2	2 1/8
13	2 5/8	2 3/8	2 7/8
14	2 3/4	3	3 1/2
15	2 5/8	3 1/4	3 5/8
16	3 1/8	3 3/8	4
17	3 3/8	3 3/8	3 3/4
18	3 3/8	3 1/2	3 5/8
19	3 1/2	3 5/8	4
20	3 3/8	3 3/4	4
21-25	3 3/8	3 3/4	4 1/8
26-30	3 3/4	4	4
31-40	3 5/8	4 1/8	4 1/2
41-50	3 1/2	4 1/8	4 3/8
51-60	3 3/4	4	4 1/4
61-65	3 3/8	4	4 5/8
66-70	3 3/8	4 1/8	4 7/8
Over 70	3 5/8	4 1/4	5

Table 1.4 Stretched Japanese penis circumference at various ages in Nakamura (1964) study.

Age (years)	Length (inches)		
	16%	Average	84%
0	1	1 1/8	1 3/8
1	1	1 1/4	1 3/8
2	1 1/8	1 1/4	1 1/2
3	1 1/8	1 3/8	1 1/2
4	1 1/4	1 3/8	1 1/2
5	1 1/4	1 1/2	1 5/8
6	1 1/4	1 1/2	1 5/8
7	1 3/8	1 1/2	1 5/8
8	1 1/4	1 1/2	1 3/4
9	1 1/4	1 1/2	1 3/4
10	1 1/4	1 3/8	1 7/8
11	1 1/4	1 1/2	1 5/8
12	1 1/4	1 1/2	1 3/4
13	1 1/4	1 3/4	2
14	1 1/2	1 7/8	2 3/8
15	2	1 7/8	2 3/4
16	2 1/8	2 1/2	2 7/8
17	2 1/4	2 3/8	3
18	2 1/4	2 7/8	2 1/2
19	2 1/4	2 3/4	3 3/8
20	2 3/8	2 3/4	3 1/4
21-25	2 1/2	2 3/4	3
26-30	2 1/2	2 3/4	3
31-40	2 5/8	2 7/8	3 1/8
41-50	2 1/4	2 7/8	3 3/8
51-60	2 3/8	2 3/4	3
61-65	2 3/8	2 3/4	3 1/4
66-70	2 1/2	2 3/4	3 1/8
Over 70	2 5/8	2 7/8	3

My Caucasian readers should use the Schonfeld and Beebe norms, which are for white Americans attempting to obtain perspective on their own stretched penis size or the size of the penises of their male children. Asian and Asian-American readers should employ the Japanese norms, since Asians tend to have smaller penises than Caucasians. There are apparently no African or African-American norms for boys and adolescents. However, Chapter 4 indicates that African-American adult men tend to have larger penises than white adult men.

The studies in the United States and Japan assessing penis growth converge to several generalizations. One is that in proportion to body weight the infant has the largest penis he will ever have. His penis may be 1" long when he weighs 8 lbs. but it is not going to be 20" long when he is 160 lbs. A second generalization is that penis size increases very little from birth to pre-adolescence. A third generalization is that there is a dramatic penis growth in early to mid adolescence. A fourth generalization is that penis growth seems ordinarily to be virtually completed by late adolescence.

I determined the ratio of stretched penis length as presented in Table 1.1 to average body weight from birth to 18 years of age. The largest ratio of .21 was at birth. The ratios decreased until the lowest of .03 at age 12. The ratios started increasing at age 13.

The period of puberty is very important in understanding sex organ growth and sexual development more generally. Schonfeld and Beebe found the average testicle size increased only 32% from the second 6 months of life to 10 years of age. In contrast to this relatively slow growth in 9+ years, there

was an increase of 1,238% from age 10 to age 15. The testicles of the average 15-year-old-boy are over 12 times larger
than those of the average 10-year-old boy.

Tanner (1962) proposed five stages of puberty that are
frequently cited in the medical literature. In stage 1, there is
no pubic hair and the penis and testes are small. In stage 2, the
testicles become larger and a small amount of pubic hair
begins to form near the base of the penis. In stage 3, the penis
becomes larger with further testicular growth and the pubic
hair becoming coarser. In stage 4, there is continued penis and
testicular growth and the spread of pubic hair growth becoming apparent. In stage 5, there is some additional growth of
the penis and testes and a great deal of pubic hair growth not
only in length but an extension upward and to a lesser extent
to the thighs. Some boys appear to have a smaller penis at
stage 5 than stage 4 because more of the penis is covered by
pubic hair.

PRACTICAL IMPLICATIONS

It is apparent from both the American and the Japanese age norms, that the greatest variability in penis size is during the period of puberty and early- to mid-adolescence (11 to 16 years). This is because in this age range we have boys who have reached puberty and those who have not reached puberty. It is not unusual for a 14 year old boy to have feelings of inferiority because his genitals are much smaller than some of his peers, who have in addition been blessed with some facial hair, lower voices, and acne. In the vast majority of such cases the situation will change within the next year. If, however, there are no indications of the beginning of puberty by age 14, a visit to the family doctor is indicated. The family doctor will probably either give reassurance that puberty will come soon or initiate testosterone or some sort of hormone treatment.

Tables 1.1, 1.2, 1.3, and 1.4 provide rough guidelines to gauge how the size of a boy's penis compares to that of other boys his age. If stretched penis length or circumference are less than the 10th percentile, this does not necessarily mean cause for serious concern, but it may be well to bring the matter to the attention of his family doctor or pediatrician.

CHAPTER 2

WHAT IS AVERAGE? WHAT IS BIG? WHAT IS SMALL?

With most human characteristics, such as IQ and height, the vast majority of persons have positions closely surrounding the average and the further we go in either direction the more uncommon or rare the occurrence becomes. Such appears to be the situation with respect to penis size.

PENIS SIZE GIVEN WITH APPARENTLY NO MEASUREMENT TAKEN

Table 2.1 shows the average penis length, diameter, and circumference stated by authors of American books and journal articles on sexual behavior. The authors of these books and articles did not state how they arrived at these averages. Most of them probably did not use systematic measurement, but based their opinions on informal observations, word of mouth, or what they had previously read. On the basis of Table 2.1 it is apparent that the estimates provided by these authors do not vary greatly. Using these estimates, we would think that the average American man has a penis that is about 3 1/2" long when flaccid and about 6" long when erect. It also would appear that the average American man has a penis that when flaccid is about 1 1/8" in diameter and when erect about 1 1/2" in diameter.

Table 2.1 Average penis size in inches as given by books and journal articles on human sexuality

Study	Length flaccid	Length erect	Diameter flaccid	Diameter erect
Stone & Stone (1953)	3 3/4	5 3/4	1	1 1/2
Gilbaugh (1993)		6		1 1/8
Reed (1996)				
Ard (1970)		5 3/4		
Green (1975)	3 3/4	5 7/8	1 1/8	1 3/8
Jones, Shamberg & Byer (1985)	3 1/2	6	1 1/4	1 1/2
Danoff (1993)	4	6	1 1/4	
Van De Velde (1957)	3 3/4	5 7/8	1 1/4	1 1/2
Katchadourian, Lunde & Trotter (1979)	3 1/2	6	1 1/4	1 1/2
Hawton (1985)	3 1/2	6		
Zilbergeld (1992)		5 3/4		
McCary (1979)	3 1/2	6	1 1/4	1 1/2
Fenwick & Pellard (1978)	3 3/4	6 1/4		
Ortiz (1989)			1 1/4	1 1/2
McCarthy (1977)	3 1/4	6	1	1 1/2
Taguchi (1985)	3 1/2	6		1 1/2
Katchadourian & Lunde (1975)	3 1/2	6	1 1/4	1 1/2
Reuben (1971)		6		
Diamond (1975)	3 3/4	5 7/8	1 1/8	1 3/8
Mendens Krop (1997)		5 7/8		
Rowan (1982)	3 7/8	6 1/8	1 1/8	1 1/2
Renshaw (1995)		6		
Engel (1995)		6		
Golderson & Anderson (1986)		6	1	1 1/2
Meeks & Heit (1984)	3 3/4	6		

15

The fact that the average size penises stated by books on sex do not differ greatly suggests that the authors may know what they are talking about. We cannot, however, be absolutely certain of this. It is possible that authors tend to state what others have written before them or what is regarded as average in folklore, casual conversation, and street-talk, which is usually "6 inches." When your author was a teenager, a young man, and a middle-aged man, the average he has heard has almost always been "6 inches" - seldom 5 1/2" or 5 3/4" or 6 1/4" or 6 1/2". It is almost always stated as "6 inches." To exaggerate a bit for emphasis, 6 inches is regarded as synonymous with an erect penis. How many erect penises have the experts who provide these sorts of estimates seen? Most men seldom see an erect penis other than their own. The number of erect adult penises that women see is quite variable, but most authors of books on sexology are men. Most sexologists who have written these books have not actually observed patients having sex. Even fewer have measured penises.

FLACCID PENIS SIZE AS MEASURED BY RESEARCHERS

Table 2.2 provides the smallest, 16th percentile, average, 84th percentile, and largest adult flaccid length and diameter as measured by researchers in various countries. On the basis of the objective measurement of researchers, it appears that the average white man has a flaccid penis that is 3 1/2" long and 1 1/8" in diameter.

16

Table 2.2 Flaccid author-measured adult penis length, circumference, and diameter in inches (table compiled by present author)

Authors and reference	Subjects	Length					Diameter				
		smallest	16th	average	84th	largest	smallest	16th	average	84th	largest
Loeb (1899)	50 Germans	2 7/8		3 3/4		4 1/2	1	1 1/8	1 1/8		1 1/4
Farkas (1971)	177 Czechs	1 7/8	2 3/8	2 7/8	3 1/4	4 3/8	1	1 1/8	1 1/4	1 3/8	1 1/2
Damon et al (1990)	50 Frenchmen	3 1/2	4 3/8	5 3/8			1	1 1/4	1 3/8	1 3/8	
Ajmani et al (1980)	320 Nigerians	2 7/8	3 1/4	3 5/8			1	1 1/8	1 1/4		1 3/8
Chaurasia & Singh (1974)	111 East Indians	2	2 5/8	2 7/8	3 1/4	3 5/8	7/8	1 1/8	1 1/8	1 1/4	1 3/8
Nedoma & Freund (1961)	252 Czechs: 126 homosexuals	2 7/8	3 3/8	3 7/8			1	1 1/8	1 1/4		
	126 heterosexuals	2 1/2	2 7/8	3 3/8			7/8	1	1 1/8		
Wilkins (1965)	Americans			3 1/8						1 1/4	
Wessells (1996)	80 Americans	2	2 1/2	3 1/2	4 1/2	6 1/8	3/4	1	1 1/4	1 3/8	1 5/8

Donald I. Templer, Ph.D.

STRETCHED PENIS SIZE AS MEASURED BY RESEARCHERS

Table 2.3 contains the smallest, 16th percentile, average, 84th percentile, and largest stretched penis length and diameter as measured by researchers in four different studies. Stretched penis length was used first by Shonfeld and Beebe (1942) and by subsequent authors as a measure of erect penis length. Schonfeld and Beebe found that stretched average penis length and erect average penis length were an almost identical 5 1/4". However, the stretched penis length of 3 3/4" for the 62 Canadian men must certainly be an underestimate of erect penis length. A reasonable statement seems to be that stretched penis length provides a minimum estimate of erect penis length.

Table 2.3 Stretched author-measured adult penis length and circumference in inches (table compiled by present author)

Authors and reference	Subjects	smallest	Length 16%	average	84%	largest
Schonfeld & Beebe (1942)	54 Americans ages 20-25		5 1/8			
Siminoski & Bain (1993)	62 Adult Canadians	2 3/8	3 1/8	3 3/4	4 1/4	5 1/4
Nakamura (1961)	184 Adult Japanese		3 3/8	3 3/4	4 1/4	
Wessells et al (1996)	80 Americans	3	3 7/8	4 7/8	6	7 1/2

ERECT PENIS AS MEASURED BY RESEARCHERS

The most scientific and objective way of determining the size of erect penises is for the researcher to do the measuring. There are only two studies in which author-measured penis size is reported. Smallest, largest, and average penis size based on these two studies is contained in Table 2.4. In both of these studies erection was produced by injection.

The study of Wessells, Lue, and McAninch (1996) is especially important for two reasons: (1) It is one of only two studies that provides researcher-measured erect state; (2) it is the only study that provides both researcher measured erect state and researcher-measured stretched state. These authors provided the relationship between both of these measures as contained in Figure 2.1. The high correspondence between stretched and erect penis size provides credence to the previous research that has used stretched penis length as an index of erect penis length. It should be noted, however, that stretched length was 1/4" less than erect length and confirms the suspicion that stretched length is a little less than erect length, 4 7/8" and 5 1/8", respectively, in the Wessells et al. study. In the da Ros et al. (1984) study the average erect penis was 5 3/4". Thus the two studies that are of the greatest scientific quality in penis measurement indicate that the average erect penis is less than the 6" that many people believe is the average length.

Table 2.4 Erect author-measured adult penis length and circumference in inches (table compiled by present author)

Authors and reference	Length			Diameter			
	Smallest 16%	average	largest 84%	Smallest 16%	average	84%	largest
Wessells et al (1996) 80 Americans	4	5 1/8	6 1/4	1 1/8	1 1/2	1 3/4	2
da Ros et al (1994) 50 Caucasian Brazilians	3 1/2	5 3/4	7 1/2	1	1 3/8		1 3/4

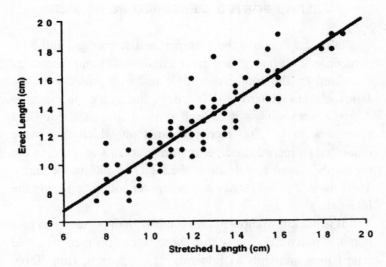

Figure 2.1 Relationship between stretched length and erect length.
(provided by Wessels, Lue & McAninch, 1996)

Donald I. Templer, Ph.D.

SELF-REPORTED MEASURED PENIS SIZE

Table 2.5 contains the 16th percentile, average, and 84th percentile adult flaccid and erect length and circumference as measured by the subjects in three research projects. In the Jamison and Gebhard (1988) article, the data of the famous Alfred Kinsey study 4 decades ago was analyzed. Kinsey and associates gave 3,500 men postcards on which they were requested to record their penis measurements and return the postcards. About two thirds of the men did mail in the cards. The Edwards (1997) study was computer conducted using the Internet.

It is not known how many men had an opportunity to participate, but we do know that there were 566 men who did report measurements to Edwards. It is apparent from Table 2.4 that these measurements tend to be larger than those provided by sexology authorities, larger than penises measured by researchers, and much larger than stretched penises measured by researchers. On the other hand, in the Internet report of students at University of California San Francisco, the self-measured erect penis length was only 5 1/8". A reasonable generalization seems to be that we can't have confidence in the accuracy of men's reports about the size of their penis.

Table 2.5 Self-measured adult flaccid and erect penis length and circumference in inches (table compiled by present author)

Authors and Reference	Subjects	Length						Diameter					
		flaccid			erect			flaccid			erect		
		16%	average	84%	16th	average	84th	16th	average	84th	16th	average	84th
Jamison & Gebhard (1988)	2625 Kinsey study Americans	3 1/4	3 7/8	4 5/8	3 1/2	6 1/4	7	1	1 1/4	1 3/8	1 1/4	1 1/2	1 3/4
Edwards (1997)	566 Americans on Internet	2 1/8	3 3/8	4 1/2	5	6 3/8	7 3/4				1 1/4	1 5/8	1 7/8
Internet (1997)	60 American College Students					5 1/8						1 1/2	

Donald I. Templer, Ph.D.

INTEGRATION OF ABOVE DESCRIBED RESEARCH

How does one integrate the pronouncements of authorities, self-measured penis size, researcher-measured flaccid penis size, researcher-measured erect penis size, and researcher-measured stretched penis size? Do we know the exact average penis size of men in the United States? Unless we go door-to-door with a tape measure or ruler, we will never know the real average. Nevertheless, we will attempt some "educated guesses." It is likely that the commonly given average of a 6" erect is an overestimate. I would say that the average Caucasian man has an erect penis of about 5 1/2" in length; that a man with a 6 1/4" penis could be fairly certain he is large, and that a man with a 4 3/4" penis can be fairly certain he is small. Most men have flaccid penises between 3" and 4" long. The average man has a flaccid penis about 1 1/8" in diameter and an erect penis about 1 3/8" in diameter. A man with an erect penis diameter of 1 3/4" can feel fairly certain he is large. A man with an erect penis diameter of 1" can feel fairly certain that he is small. Virtually all men, however, can find a woman who thinks that his penis is just right for her.

A fact that authorities on sex have established is that penises that are larger while flaccid expand less while erect, and penises that are smaller while flaccid expand more while erect. This fact makes many men unnecessarily believe that they have a small penis on the basis of locker room observations when they really are average or even above average in the erect state. Most men seldom see the erect penis of other men. Simple counseling about such matters may be very help-

24

ful for men whose penises are small while flaccid but not small when erect.

The majority of recognized authorities on sexual behavior maintain that a substantial percentage of men feel inadequate about the size of their penis. With some men this is a function of actually having a small penis. With other men it may have to do with the locker room observation of flaccid penises described above. Also, when a man looks down on his penis it appears smaller than that of the same size penis on a man 10' away. This may especially be the case if one is obese. Perhaps another factor is that most men don't know the size of the erect penises of their sex partner's previous sex partners. Even a man with a large penis may have the thought that his lover may have on a previous occasion or occasions had a larger penis in her vagina. If a survey of men were determined and the respondents were all honest, the vast majority of men would probably acknowledge that they wish they had a larger penis.

There is apparently only one study that correlated penis girth with penis length. Figure 2.2 contains the "scatter plot" provided by Edwards (1997). Each dot represents the length and circumference of the penis of one man. The scatter plot tells us that there is a tendency for men with longer penises to have thicker penises. This should not surprise us and is consistent with common sense. Nevertheless, the relationship is not a strong one.

Although extremely large penises are very uncommon, they do receive considerable attention, especially if the man who possesses the huge penis is famous. There are a number of famous men who reportedly had an extraordinarily large

25

Donald I. Templer, Ph.D.

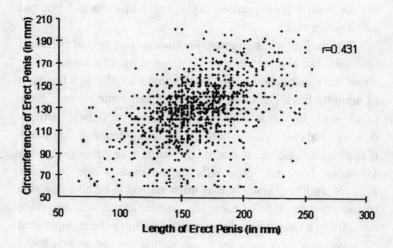

Figure 2.2 Scatter gram of erect penis circumference versus erect penis length (from Edwards, 1997).

penis. We will probably never know to what extent these stories are based on fact and to what extent they are based on myth. Rutledge (1996) discussed some of these famous men:

FAMOUS MEN,
ALL REPUTEDLY VERY WELL-ENDOWED

1. **Lord Byron** (1788-1824), English poet

His reputation as a libertine prevented him from being buried in Poet's Corner at Westminster Abbey, and he was interred instead in a small church near Nottingham, England. In 1938, 114 years after his death, the burial vault was opened, and Byron's body was found to be well-preserved with the features easily recognizable. One observer noted: "His sexual organ shewed quite abnormal development."

2. **Errol Flynn** (1909-1959), U.S. actor

He was obsessively proud of the size of his penis and, according to Truman Capote, took it out of his pants at a party one night and tried to play "You Are My Sunshine" on the piano with it.

3. **Frank Sinatra** (1915-1998), U.S. singer

When his second wife, actress Ava Gardner, was asked what she saw in the "one-hundred-twenty-pound runt," she replied, "Well, there's only ten pounds of Frank, but there's one hundred and ten pounds of (penis)!"

Donald I. Templer, Ph.D.

4. **Aristotle Onassis** (1906-1975). Greek shipping magnate

He sometimes referred to his huge penis as "the secret of my success" and once dragged an obnoxious reporter into the men's room to prove just how well-endowed he was. Maria Callas told a friend, "When I met Aristo, so full of life, I became a different woman."

5. **Milton Berle** (1908-2002), U.S. entertainer

Berle's reputation for being well-endowed was so well-known that he was challenged to a bet by a stranger who claimed his penis was bigger than Berle's. Berle took the man into a nearby rest room to settle the wager; but despite goading from his friends to show off the whole thing, Berle would pull out only enough to win the bet.

6. **Charlie Chaplin** (1889-1977), U.S. filmmaker and actor

He cheerfully referred to himself as "the Eighth Wonder of the World."

7. **Fatty Arbuckle** (1887-1933), U.S. silent-screen comedian

In 1921, after a three-day wild party that left the twelfth floor of San Francisco's Hotel St. Francis in shambles, the 300-pound comedian was charged with manslaughter in the death of a young starlet he had allegedly raped. The girl had died of peritonitis and a ruptured bladder, leading to rumors about Arbuckle's supposedly gargantuan endowment. After two mistrials Arbuckle was finally acquitted of the murder, but by then Paramount had canceled his contract, and his career was finished.

8. **Charles II** (1630-1685), king of England

He was nicknamed "Old Rowley" after a studhorse he owned. It was sometimes joked that his scepter and his penis were of equal length.

9. **Gary Cooper** (1901-1961), U.S. actor

Cooper's reputation for being exceptionally well-endowed helped accelerate his notoriety as one of Hollywood's most prodigious lovers. When Tallulah Bankhead was asked why she was leaving New York for Hollywood in the 1940s, she said it was "to (have sexual intercourse with) that divine Gary Cooper."

10. **John Dillinger** (1902-1934), U.S. Bank Robber

For years it was rumored that his penis was an incredible 12 inches long when flaccid, 20 to 22 inches long when erect. However, one eyewitness to Dillinger's autopsy later testified that the outlaw had a normal endowment.

11. **Jack London** (1876-1916) U.S. writer

The handsome, muscular writer was often referred to as "the Stallion" by his friends.

12. **Aldo Ray** (1926-1991), U.S. Actor

After making a name for himself as a character actor in such films as *Miss Sadie Thompson* and *God's Little Acre*, his Hollywood career started to slide in the early '60s. He then jumped into the burgeoning porno movie business, where his husky good looks and extra-large endowment helped him find a whole new audience of admirers.

13. **Henri de Toulouse-Latrec** (1864-1901), French artist

Crippled in adolescence, he never grew taller than 5 foot 1, but his genitals were unusually large, even for a man of normal size. Referring to his squat body and enormous penis, he described himself as "a coffeepot with a big spout." Friends sometimes referred to him as *verges a pattes*: "a walking penis."

PRACTICAL IMPLICATIONS

Practical implications have already been described in this chapter but will here be reiterated. First of all, men have been made to feel inferior because 6" has been given as the average penis length. The scientific evidence indicates that the Caucasian average is somewhat less than this. Many men also feel inferior because of the size of their flaccid penis. Men should know that the differences in erect penis size are less than what might be presumed from locker room observation of flaccid penis size. Flaccid penises that are compressed like an accordion extend more in becoming erect than penises that hang down. A man with a large penis is often referred to as "hung." However, the man who appears to be "hung" in the flaccid state may be no larger in the erect state than that of the man whose penis appears shriveled up in the flaccid state.

It is *very* common for men with penises that are small, but not abnormally small, to be very concerned about their endowment. Simple counseling is often quite effective. These men should be told that many women prefer small penises and that many women have no size preference. If their current sex partner prefers a large penis, there are sexual positions described in Chapter 6 that can often satisfactorily compensate for the limited size. Murtaugh (1989), a family doctor in Australia, described 3 cases in which he provided effective counseling for men with concerns about their somewhat smaller than average penises:

Donald I. Templer, Ph.D.

Three case histories

Case 1: Mr. J, aged 31

Mr. J, aged 31, an accountant, presented for a check-up mainly because he was getting married and wanted to know "if he was fit for married life." Apart from the usual childhood illnesses he claimed to be always very healthy and had no significant adverse family history.

He seemed rather shy and introspective and upon direct questioning about any possible concerns about his forthcoming marriage stated that he was "'rather anxious about whether he would be a good husband and father."

On confrontation about the reason for such a statement he revealed a history of mumps at 16 years when one of his testicles was affected. He also talked about concerns about his "masculinity" and about the size of his penis which he considered was probably too small. Furthermore, he revealed that his two attempts at intercourse with his fiancée were most unsatisfactory, resulting in premature ejaculation. He felt very embarrassed about his problem which he could not discuss with his fiancée.

Examination revealed normal external genitalia including normal testes and a penis three inches (7.5 cm) long with a circumference of three and a half inches (nine cm).

Appropriate counseling with reassurance, based on this examination, appeared to give him considerable relief of mind.

Case 2: Mr. T, aged 36

Mr. T, aged 36, a member of a religious community, presented for a check-up after deciding to leave the religious life and "seek his fame and fortune in the secular world." He described a desire to find a suitable woman, get married, and lead a normal family life.

Despite an initial evasiveness, his concern about sexual inadequacy was obvious. When the subject was raised discreetly he talked about his concern whether his penis was adequate for normal sexual function and satisfaction for the opposite sex. He offered the information that his erect penis was 12 cm long.

Examination revealed a relatively small penis just less than 3 inches long (seven cm). He was reassured that there were many millions of men in the world with similar dimensions who enjoyed a normal sex life.

Donald I. Templer, Ph.D.

Case 3: Mr. B, aged 31

Mr. B, aged 25, a teacher and champion sportsman, had presented several times over a period of about eight weeks for relatively trivial complaints, mainly of a musculosketal nature and feelings of tiredness and lethargy. Soon afterwards a hand delivered letter contained the following information:

Dear Doctor,

I hope I can take a couple of your precious minutes to discuss a subject that's been a major worry for me for a long time. It is very awkward and most embarrassing letter to write.

I want to ask you if anything can be done in relation to the size of one's penis. You're probably thinking this is the wish of many a young man; however, I do believe I have a special case.

All I want to know is can anything be done at all, no matter how drastic the measure needs to be? It has got to a stage that is wrecking my whole life. Many times when I let it get the better of me, my self concept, my thoughts on the future are almost zero — completely negative.

It is a constant worry and I know it restricts my total personality. I know it does not directly affect my "sexual performance" but I wonder now at 25 whether I will ever be able to accept a wife. I know many would say it is purely a psychological thing.

Doctor, I need to know if there is any chance of doing anything to rectify what I believe is an under-

34

developed penis. Perhaps due to a lack of male hormone during puberty — I don't know.

I know the next step is examination and that will
be embarrassing but I thought if I could give you a little time to assess the situation it would be better.

He did have a relatively small penis, two and a half inches (six cm), which was just below the accepted normal range
of three to four inches. However, he did volunteer that on
erection it reached four and one half to five inches (12 cm)
which is within normal limits.

Murtagh (1989) implied that his counseling was effective
in these three cases. He did not, however, provide any follow-
up information.

CHAPTER 3

SIZE OF THE PENIS AND THE SIZE OF THE MAN

One would think that the size of a penis is highly correlated with the size of the man who possesses it. The man who is 6'4" tall usually has longer arms, hands, fingers, feet and legs than a short man. Sometimes people talk about being able to estimate the size of a man's penis by his height or his shoe size or hand size.

In spite of the fact that common sense suggests that larger men have larger penises, most of the experts in the field state that there is no relationship between the size of a man and the size of his penis. For example, Rowan (1982) said, "There is no relationship between penis size and any other body measurement such as height, arm length, or nose size." My analysis of the scientific evidence shows that these experts are wrong.

What does the scientific evidence indicate? The research in which measurements were taken in a systematic fashion and subjected to proper statistical analysis supports the contention that there is a positive but modest relationship between penis size and size of the man.

Fisher (1964) determined the relationship between flaccid penis length and height in 50 German men. He found that taller men tended to have larger penises. In Figure 4.1 each dot shows the height and flaccid penis length of a man. The penis of the shortest man was 3 1/8" long. The penis of the tallest man was 4 3/8" long. Figure 3.1 shows, however, that there are tall men with short penises and short men with long penises.

Figure 3.1 suggests that there does not seem to be much difference in flaccid penis length of short and medium height men. However, the penises of the 15 tallest men are definitely more likely to be over 4" long than are those of the other men. As illustrated in Table 3.1, 60% of the 15 tallest men but only 21% of the other 35 men had flaccid penises over 4" long.

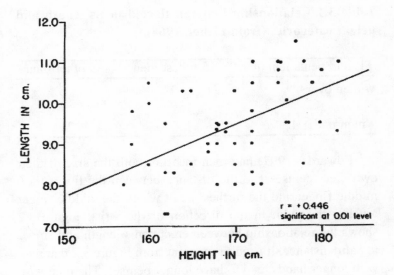

Figure 3.1 Relationship between height and length of penis.
(from Fischer, 1964).

In the data presented by Fisher there was no relationship between height and penis circumference. Perhaps this is because height is a measure of length rather than girth. It is possible that penis circumference may correlate with a measure of body thickness, such as wrist size, but research of this sort has apparently not been carried out.

Suminoski and Bain (1993) reported a low but significant correlation between penis size and height. They also found a low but significant correlation between the size of the men's penises and their shoe size.

39

Table 3.1 Relationship between flaccid penis length and height categories (from Fisher, 1964).

Flaccid penis length	15 tallest men	35 other men
# men over 4"	9	6
# men under 4"	6	21

Edwards (1997) had men measure both the size of their own erect penises and the distance between the tip of their middle finger and the furthest point where the middle finger touches the palm in the direction of the wrist. Figure 3.2 shows the relationship between erect penis length and finger to palm distance. It is quite apparent from Figure 3.2 that men with longer hands tend to have longer penises. The men with longer penises also tended to have a larger shoe size. Shoe size, however, was not as strongly related to penis size as was hand size.

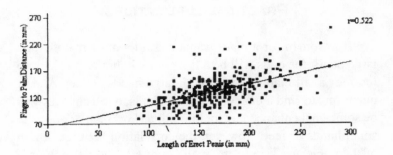

Figure 3.2 Relationship between hand size and length of erect penis (from Edwards, 1997).

The research of Ajmani, Jain, and Saxena (1985) showed a very small relationship between height and penis size of Nigerian medical students. Flaccid penis length was 3.18" for the 110 men less than 5'6" tall, 3.20" for the 150 men between 5'6" and 5'9" tall, and 3.25" for the 60 men over 5'9" tall. Thus the men in the tallest group had penises only 1/16th" longer than the men in the two shorter groups. The circumferences for the three groups were almost identical, 3.46", 3.47", and 3.48", respectively.

Apparently the positive correlation between penis length and body size exists even at birth. A study found that penis length of newborn Israeli infants was positively and significantly associated with birth length and birth weight (Flatau, Josefsberg, Reisner, Bialik, & Laron, 1975).

41

PRACTICAL IMPLICATIONS

If a woman (or a man) wants to find a male mate with a large penis, the odds will be a little more in her or his favor to look for a tall man or a man with large hands or feet. And, if one wants to find a man with a small penis, one's chances will be somewhat enhanced by looking for a short man or one with small hands or feet. However, the correlation between length of the penis and size of the man is not a high one. Asking a man the size of his penis may be a better way of determining size, although it should be borne in mind that men are not always honest in this regard. A still better way of determining the size of a man's penis is to actually look!

CHAPTER 4

RACIAL DIFFERENCES IN PENIS SIZE

It is part of American folklore and stereotype that African-American men have larger penises than white American males. A large percentage of Americans believe this is an established fact. Other persons are less convinced or say there is no difference. A number of jokes that white persons tell are about extraordinarily large black penises. With many white American males there are feelings of inferiority about the alleged difference. This feeling of inferiority is probably strengthened by casual observations in locker rooms and showers. This may be in part a function of African-American men having less of a size difference between the flaccid and erect state. The white man with the 3" flaccid penis sees that the black man with the 6 inch flaccid penis and assumes, that since his own is 6" erect, the Black man's penis is 12" when erect, when indeed it may be more like 7" long when erect. Nevertheless, it probably is a correct statement that, on the average, black penises tend to be larger than white penises.

Gebhard and Johnson (1979) presented information on comparative penis sizes of black and white men on the basis of Alfred Kinsey's famous research. Since measurement was done by the subjects and since self-measurement tends to be larger than researcher measurement, we can't have confidence that the penis sizes provided are accurate. Nevertheless, there is no reason to believe that either the black or white subjects were more prone to report inaccurate measurements. Table 4.1 contains the percentage of black and white men with larger and smaller penis size. Both length and circumference and flaccid and erect measurements are given. The greatest differences are with flaccid penis length. There are almost three times the percentage of black than white men who have a flaccid penis over 4 1/2" long. There are almost five times the percentage of white than black men who have a flaccid penis 3" long or less. White men are less "inferior" to black men in circumference and when the penis is erect.

Table 4.1 Comparison of penis size of Black and White men. (From Gebhard & Johnson, 1979; table constructed by present author).

Penis Size	% Black Men	% White Men
Length		
Flaccid penis length		
over 4 1/2 inches	32.3%	11.3%
3 inches or less	3.4%	16.2%
Erect penis length		
over 7 inches	16.6%	7.6%
4 3/4 inches or less	0%	3.3%
Circumference		
Flaccid penis circumference (3.14 times diameter)		
Over 4 inches	30.6%	21.2%
2 1/4 inch or less	3.4%	4.0%
Erect penis circumference (3.14 times diameter)		
Over 5 1/2 inches	23.7%	19.5%
3 3/4 inches or less	3.6%	6.4%

Donald I. Templer, Ph.D.

Rushton (1995) presented a very informative table based upon the World Health Program on AIDS Specifications and Guidelines for Condom Procurement. Although we don't know how the measurements were taken, it is readily apparent that there are distinctly different erect penis length distributions for Thai men, American white men, and African-American men. About 80% of the Thai men had erect penises from 4" to 5 7/8" long. About 80% of white American men had erect penises from 5" to 6 7/8" long. And, about 80% of African-American men had erect penises from 5 7/8" to 7 1/8" long. The erect circumference distributions of white Americans and African-Americans were similar. The Thai men, however, tended to have lesser girth. Fifty-three percent of the Thai men, but only 18% of the white men and 13% of the black men, had an erect penis circumference of 4 7/8" or less. It should be no surprise, then, that the World Health Organization recommends different size condoms for men of Asian, European, and African ancestry.

Grady and Tanfer (1994) reported that black men who used condoms were five times more likely to report condom breakage than men of other races who used condoms. Grady and Tanfer said that they didn't know how to explain this finding. However, I suggest that the breakage could be caused by the larger average penis size of African-American men.

There is considerable evidence that Asian men on the average have smaller penises than White men. Condoms manufactured in Japan to be sold in the United States are larger than those manufactured to be sold in Japan. Condoms manufactured in the United States to be sold in Japan are smaller than those manufactured to be sold in the United States.

46

It is apparent from comparing the American and Japanese penis averages in Chapter 1 that the American stretched penises tend to be appreciably larger. The American penises are roughly 25% larger than the Japanese penises in girth across the age range, and the American penis length averages tend to be over 1 1/2 times that of the Japanese average during childhood and about 40% longer during the adolescent and early adult years.

It appears that Asian women have smaller vaginas than American women. Women in Thailand complain about the American female condoms being too large for their anatomy. American military personnel during the Vietnam War era reported that Vietnamese women have smaller vaginas than white women. Also, quite a few Vietnamese prostitutes refused to have sexual intercourse with American men, black or white, who had exceptionally large penises.

In the research of Edwards (1997) cited in Chapter 2, the reported average for the self measured erect penis was 6 3/8" for the black men, 6 3/8" for the Caucasian men, 5 3/8" for the Hispanic men, and 5 1/2" for the East Asian (Chinese, Japanese, Korean and Vietnamese) men. Edwards reported that the black and Caucasian groups still had statistically greater penis size than the Asian and Hispanic men when height was controlled for. In contrast to previous studies, there was no difference between black and Caucasian penis sizes, but there were not many black men included in the study. Hispanic persons have more in common with respect to language than to ethnic ancestry. Most Mexican-Americans have at least as much Indian as Spanish sanguenity. Physical anthropologists tell us that Native-Americans are fundamen-

Donald I. Templer, Ph.D.

tally Oriental people. Hispanics in the Caribbean region are more likely to have African ancestry.

Rushton and Bogaert (1987) reported:

"The ethnographic record [e.g., a French Army Surgeon (1898/1972), a 30-year specialist in genitourinary diseases] makes references to numerous anatomical distinctions which show a similar pattern of Whites being between Blacks and Orientals. These include the placement of female genitals (Orientals front and high; Blacks back and low); angle and texture of erection (Orientals parallel to body and stiff, Blacks at right angles to body and flexible); salient buttocks, breasts, and muscularity (Orientals least, Blacks most); and size of genitalia (Orientals least, Blacks most). We averaged the ethnographic data on erect penis and found the means to approximate: Orientals, 4 to 5.5 in. in length and 1.25 in. in diameter; Caucasians, 5.5 to 6 in. in length and 1.5 in. in diameter; Blacks, 6.25 to 8 in. in length and 2 in. in diameter. Women were proportionate to men, with Orientals having smaller vaginas and Blacks larger ones, relative to Caucasians. Clitoral size differed in length: in European women, 1.2 in.: in African women, 2 in variations were noted: In the French West Indies, the size of the penis and vagina covaried with amount of Black admixture: Arab men, who were often mixed with Black, had larger penises than Europeans."

Choi, Cho and Xin (1994) reported that the standard penile prosthesis made for American men is too large for the Oriental penis. They stated that these devises are especially

48

too large in diameter. Oh, Choi, and Kim (1990) also reported that the American made prostheses are too large for the smaller penises of Korean men.

Rushton (1992) had Canadian white and Oriental college students rank the size of genitals as a function of race. Both the white and the Oriental students believed that blacks have larger sexual organs than whites and that whites have larger sex organs than Orientals. One must bear in mind that these assessments are merely opinions that could be biased by stereotypes. On the other hand, these opinions do mesh with other evidence.

In this chapter the Asian men referred to are primarily East Asian ("Oriental") men. However, the unsystematic impressions stated in the literature are that men from the Indian subcontinent also tend to have penises smaller than those of American and European men. As is contained in Chapter 2, Chaurasia and Singh (1974) measured the flaccid penis of 111 medical students in India. The penis lengths ranged from 2" to 3 5/8" with an average of 2 7/8". The 16th percentile was 2 5/8" and the 84th percentile was 3 1/4". The circumference ranged from 2 3/4" to 4 3/8" with an average of 3 1/2". The 16th percentile was 3 1/8", and the 84th percentile was 3 3/4". The length of flaccid penises of Indian men seems to differ more from those of American and European men than the circumference measurements.

Chapter 2 cited research of Ajmani, Jain, and Saxina (1985) with Nigerian men who provided an average flaccid penis of 3 1/4", which seems to be shorter than that of the average African-American man. Perhaps the differences are a function of measurement technique, nutrition, or gene pool. It is noteworthy that the Nigerian men were of considerably shorter height than the typical African-American man. For the former, 34% were less than 5'6" tall, 47% between 5'6" and 5'9" tall, and only 19% more than 5'9" tall.

It is of interest to note that there is an accumulation of evidence that African-American boys and girls reach puberty at an earlier age than white boys and girls (Westney, Jenkins, Butts, & Williams, 1984). Westney et al. (1984) reported that although 12 1/2 years of age is when the average white boy shows the beginning of penis growth, 33% of 10-year-old African-Americans and 60% of 11-year-old African-Americans studied had reached this stage. White Americans reach puberty before Asian Americans.

Phillip, DeBoer, Pilpel, Karplus, and Sofer (1996) compared the penis size and clitoris size of Jewish and Arabic Bedouin newborns in Israel. The study was based on the observations of one of the authors that Arab infant girls have larger clitoris size than Jewish girls. This impression was confirmed in that the Arab and Jewish girls had an average clitoris length of 6.61 millimeters and 5.87 millimeters, respectively. The penis sizes of the boys were 37.1 and 36.1 millimeters, respectively, a difference that is in the same direction but quite small. It has been maintained that Arab men, especially those with Negroid features, tend to have large penises. There has been, however, apparently no scientific study that has compared the penis size of adult Arab males with that of other men.

Goto (1997) did not present any systemic data analysis but did discuss the issue of Asian penis size with a number of different people, some of whom believe that Asian men have smaller penises and some of whom say that Asian penises do not differ in size from those of white men. Here is what Goto wrote:

"Through my research, I found one Asian male, a Japanese American, late 20's, who said he has a 7-inch penis. He even offered to show it to me, to which I immediately declined. He boasted that he gained instant notoriety after dating someone in the Los Angeles Asian American Community.

"'Girls would point at me,' he said. 'It was a pretty big ego boost!'

"A Vietnamese American Male, early 20's, admitted he was 'below' the average of 6 inches. Asked if he was ever concerned about the length of his penis, he simply answered, 'No.'

"A Japanese American female, early 20's, said she has been with two Asian men: a half Filipino, half Chinese in his mid-20's, and a Japanese in his mid-20's.

"With the 6-inch rule in mind, she said, 'Okay, let me think about this. I have to think how long six inches is. Well, I guess they were average. Yeah, they were about average.'

"I assumed that the women's accounts of penis size to be more reliable than the men's. However, while conducting my research, a homosexual Caucasian man - we'll call him Brian - in his late 30's, volunteered some information.

"'I would say that from a purely statistical point of view, [the myth of the Asian penis being smaller] is basically true,' he said. 'However, the smallest I've experienced was on a Caucasian.'

"Brian said that he has dated about 40 Asian men and about 15 to 20 Caucasian men. He added that he prefers Asian men to men of any other ethnicity.

"'I think that what I've found among Asian men is the absence of really 'big ones', he said. But I think if you were to put White men and Asian men on two separate bell curves, there would be a lot of overlap.

"Among two Filipino women, late 20's to early 30's, one initially said 'way above average.' Then I found out she was talking about her fiancé, who is African American. So much for that myth.

"The other woman said the Japanese man she dated was 'average.' She then added, 'I can't believe you're asking these questions!'

"Yet Donna thought the subject of this article was interesting, since most of her boyfriends have been Asian. She explained that she prefers Asian men 'because they're small.'

"Donna, who stands about 5'1", thinks 'body size' has something to do with penis size.

"'Asian men are not big,' she said, referring to their penises. 'I guess that's always why I liked Asian men. I strongly believe that that's because of their bodies. Their bodies are not big.'

"I told her the average size for all males is about 6 inches. She replied, 'Yeah. They (Asian men) are average.'

"Donna's friend, a Chinese American female, early 20's, said she currently dates African American men. She made it clear that it is 'the whole physical package' of African American men that appeals to her, not their penis size. She said she has dated one Asian man whose penis was 'about 6 1/2 inches, but it was big in circumference.'

"Asked if she was familiar with the different ethnic-specific stereotypes, she replied, 'Not all Asian men are going to have smaller penises in the same way that not all Black men have huge penises. There's exceptions to every stereotype. Just because I'm Asian doesn't mean I'm going to be passive.'

"A Chinese American female - let's call her Marilyn - in her mid-20's explained that she hadn't been with a lot of men, but that she had 'been very lucky.'

"'Every single guy has been at least 6 inches,' Marilyn said. 'They were mostly Chinese men. One was 8 inches, another was 7 inches. I guess I've been pretty lucky.'

"A Korean American male, mid-20's, recalled a conversation with his Caucasian girlfriend. He said they had just finished making love when she brought up the subject of penis size.

"'She said she had heard about the size myth, and initially she was kind of concerned,' he said. 'It was something that was in the back of her mind, before we ever made love. But after making love, she found out it wasn't a problem, that [the myth] wasn't true.'

"He said he was always a little uncomfortable with the subject of penis size because all of his friends who

were White had joked about how little Asian men's penises must be. After a while, he began to believe in the myth
himself.

"'It plays on your psyche,' he said. 'My friends used
to joke and poke fun at me and say, 'You know how Asian
men are.'

"'Back at the same college where I took Dirty 230, I
had the circumstance of being one of only about 200
Asians on campus, out of a total enrollment of about
17,000. Most of my friends, roommates, classmates, pro-
fessors, etc. were Caucasian.

"'I will never forget the experience nor the questions
I faced every day. Do you eat rice? Do you use chop-
sticks?" But those questions were nothing compared to
the graphically sexual ones I heard about Asian women.

"'I heard that Asian women are "tighter," several
acquaintances would say, in reference to the vagina.
Another reference never ceased to amaze me every time I
heard it: "I heard that Asian women's (vaginal openings)
were horizontal instead of vertical so that it would get
tighter as they spread their legs."

'You would be seriously be amazed by all the questions I have heard about Asian women in the five years I
attended that university. But back to this Asian penis
thing.

"Donna, the Columbian woman, said she dated a
Columbian man whose penis was 'so big that it hurt.'

'[The Columbian man] was someone who I could've
married,' she said. But I wouldn't marry him for many
reasons. One reason was because he (his penis) was too

big. My friends said, 'Oh, you'll get used to it.' But I never did. I couldn't stand it!"

"The woman I referred to as Marilyn admitted she doesn't particularly like sex with a man much bigger than 6 inches.

'With someone that huge, it really hurts,' she said. ' I don't think I ever want something that big inside me again.'

"One of the females I interviewed was curious as to what the consensus was on Asian penis size. I told her that the results were about average. Some bigger, some smaller, mostly average though.

"She was surprised to hear 'some bigger.' I was talking to her on the phone, but I could just imagine her eyes growing wider with amazement. She was even surprised to hear that Asian men were about average, having heard the myth of the small Asian penis as well."

Donald I. Templer, Ph.D.

PRACTICAL IMPLICATIONS

If a woman is looking for a man with a relatively large penis, her chances of finding such a man are somewhat increased by dating African-American men. A woman's chances of finding a sex partner with a small penis are somewhat increased by dating Asian men. However, there are many African-American men with small penises and many Asian men with large penises. Ethnicity can also serve as a predictor of the vaginal size of a woman with African-American, white, and Asian vaginas having the same ranking as that for penises. I doubt, however, if ethnicity is a better predictor of vaginal size than whether or not a woman has given birth to a child. It is of interest to note that it is more common for a white woman to marry an African-American man than for an African-American woman to marry a white man. It is also more common for a white man to marry an Asian woman than for a white woman to marry an Asian man. It is unusual for an Asian man to marry an African-American woman.

Many persons wish to date and marry within one's own ethnicity. If one has such a preference, it is not necessary to look for men or women outside of one's ethnicity. You can find the penis or vagina size you want either in your own or in other ethnicities.

CHAPTER 5

ABNORMALLY SMALL PENIS SIZE

Of the millions of men who have small penises, only a small percentage of them have a penis so small that it could be described as abnormal. This chapter deals primarily with rare or very unusual medical conditions that are associated with abnormally small or smaller than average penises. The section on precocious puberty deals with young boys who have adult size penises caused by medical abnormality.

MICROPENIS

In micropenis the penis is often extremely small and sometimes not much bigger than a clitoris. Micropenis can result from a number of conditions and becomes manifest at birth. There is moderately effective treatment with testosterone administration and sometimes surgery. Nevertheless, when adulthood is reached the penis is usually below average in size. It is important that micropenis be treated early in life because when adulthood is reached not much growth can be induced by hormonal means.

Van Seters and Sloh (1988) reported on an adult patient with micropenis who had a mutually gratifying heterosexual relationship. He had a one inch long penis and advertised in a national newspaper "a young man, small proportioned, wishes contact with a woman." He and the woman married and had a mutually satisfying sexual relationship. He stated:

"I think the emphasis in our lovemaking is on our
hands. We do a lot with them. She really enjoys
being caressed. What we also enjoy is oral sex.
We do try to achieve an intromission occasionally,
in a special position with a pillow under her buttocks,
but that's not the way to reach orgasm."

Money, Lehne, and Norman (1983) reported on the IQ testing of 20 patients with micropenis. The range was from 81 to 137, with an average IQ of 117. Only about 15% of the general population have an IQ of 117 or higher. The reason for such high IQs in men with such small penises are not known. Nevertheless, it is nice to learn that nature is not entirely unfair to these men in the realm of endowment.

DELAYED PUBERTY

It is sometimes difficult to differentiate "delayed puberty" in which the puberty will eventually arrive from a medical condition in which there is inadequate testosterone. The 15 year old boy with a penis the size of a ten year old could suffer psychologically and socially. Also, one can't always be certain that puberty will eventually arrive. Delayed puberty is the most common cause for a boy in his early teens having a very small penis. The usual treatment is monthly administration of testosterone for 4 to 12 months (Cronau & Brown, 1998).

DOWN'S SYNDROME

Down's syndrome is one of the most common forms of mental retardation. The patient ordinarily has a characteristic facial appearance, mild obesity, short stature, proneness to heart problems, and a life expectancy of below 60 years. Males with Down's syndrome ordinarily have below average, but not greatly so, penis size. One study found adult males with Down's Syndrome to have an average stretched penis length of 3 3/8" (Pueschel, Orson, Boylan, & Pezzullo, 1985).

KLINEFELTER'S SYNDROME

Klinefelter's syndrome occurs in 1 in 500 live male births. There is usually an extra X chromosome. A disproportionate number of persons with this disorder are mentally retarded and/or exhibit antisocial behavior. Men with Klinefelter's syndrome tend to have below average (but not greatly so) penises and testes in addition to below average facial and body hair and sometimes female type fat distribution and gynecomastia (breast development in the male).

Donald I. Templer, Ph.D.

KALLMAN'S SYNDROME

Kallman's syndrome is a disorder in which there is insufficient testosterone and a small penis and testicles. It is often associated with color blindness, inability to smell, and sometimes cleft lip and palate. The disorder tends to run in families.

PRADER-WILLI SYNDROME

In Prader-Willi syndrome, a congenital condition, features include mental retardation, insatiable hunger, massive obesity, short stature, lethargy, inactivity, irritability, increased picking of the skin, and stubbornness. In a study of 115 male cases, Greenswag (1987) reported that 92% had small penises. Also common were undescended testes, little or no body hair, and little or no facial hair.

MASSIVE OBESITY

In addition to the true size of a man's penis being concealed by fat, severely obese men sometimes have low levels of testosterone, high levels of estrogen, impotence, low sex drive, and a small penis caused by the obesity.

PRECOCIOUS PUBERTY

Precocious puberty is defined as puberty below the age of 8 in females and 10 in males. In addition to the adult size genitals, there are other indications that puberty has been reached in the male, such as facial and body hair. Medical attention is definitely needed. The cause can be a serious condition, such as an endocrine disorder or brain tumor. When no such cause can be found it is called "idiopathic" precocious puberty. In idiopathic precocious puberty and some other types, the intervention consists of reversing the abnormal hormonal situation until the normal age of puberty. It should be noted that anabolic steroid drugs used for strength and muscularity in prepubescent boys can bring about early puberty with an adult size penis. A premature puberty, regardless of cause, can result in a somewhat shorter adult height than would have been expected with a normal age puberty.

PRACTICAL IMPLICATIONS

The first person to see if you believe you or your son has an abnormally small penis is your family physician or pediatrician. He or she will make a referral to another medical specialist if this is deemed necessary. Some cases of an abnormally small penis can be helped a great deal and some can be helped very little. If the latter is the situation, counseling with a mental health practitioner such as a psychologist, psychiatrist, or social worker may be indicated.

If you suspect precocious puberty in your child, take him or her to a physician without delay. Precocious puberty can be associated with a life- threatening medical condition.

CHAPTER 6

WHAT SIZE PENISES WOMEN PREFER

The preponderance of experts on sex maintain that penis size and vagina size have no or almost no relationship to sexual pleasure and satisfaction. They tend to say that incompatibility of genital size is rare. They cite the fact that the vagina can expand sufficiently to give birth to a baby. They cite the fact that the inner two thirds of the vagina is relatively insensitive to touch. These experts have impressive credentials and a great deal of clinical experience as sexologists.

Ard (1970) said, "Basically, the female vagina is so constructed that it stretches to accommodate whatever size penis is inserted. This is practically a fool-proof arrangement as far as genital size is concerned. A man's ability to satisfy a woman in the sex act does *not* depend on the size of his penis. The sooner we get rid of this notion the better off everyone will be." Stuart (1971) asserted that "The size of a man's penis is not a central concern to a woman, who knows from experience that she is equally satisfied by any size, as long as the man wielding it knows what he's doing." Roen (1975) stated, "I can not emphasize too strongly that it is not the size of an erect penis which makes for adequate sexual response in either men or women. A woman's vagina distends only for the size of the penis which is inserted, so the dimensions of the penis make no difference to either partner." Reuben (1971) maintained that "There is no relation, whatsoever between the size of the penis - length, diameter, or any other measurement - and the ability to produce sexual orgasm in the female." McCary (1979) said, "The measurement of a perfectly functioning erect penis might vary from two inches in one man to ten inches in another, one being no less capable of coital performance than the other." Shearer and Shearer (1972) said, "Actually, the size of the penis is relatively unimportant in regard to effective sexual functioning since the vagina has nerve endings in only the outer third." They went on to say, "Therefore there is really no problem about whether a penis will be too large to be accommodated in the vagina. Basically, there is no true incompatibility, especially after the hyman has been enlarged, which occurs at the first intercourse."

Nevertheless, pleasure and pain are subjective experiences and the people who can tell us how and what they feel are those who have the experience. Whose reports do you have more faith in - the experts or the women who actually have the experiences? I listen more closely to what the women have to say.

IS SIZE IMPORTANT?

The remainder of this chapter is divided into four parts. In part A the opinions of women given in surveys are presented. Part B contains the opinions of gynecologists on the basis of their clinical experience. Part C contains miscellaneous material. The fourth part contains practical implications, including Kegel exercises.

PART A: OPINIONS OF WOMEN OBTAINED IN SURVEYS

Even though most persons who are regarded as experts in the field of sexology say penis size ordinarily is of little or no importance, when women are questioned about the matter, many women do have a preference. Some like large penises, some medium penises, and some small penises. In most of the surveys the methodology is far from perfect by scientific standards. The women were apparently not selected to be representative of American women, and we sometimes have no idea as to how they were selected; therefore, we are unable to state what percentage of American women like penises of various sizes. On the basis of the comments it would appear that these women tend to have sufficient experiences to be able to make comparisons. Women who are sexually inexperienced and women who have not had children may prefer smaller penises for their relatively smaller vaginas. Nevertheless, the statements of the women do provide us with the reasons that larger or smaller penises are preferred and the thoughts and feelings associated with the experiences.

In the Internet survey of Edwards (1997) the women were asked, "During sex how important is the length of a man's penis?" Twenty-five percent of the respondents said "very important," 58% "somewhat important," and 16% "not important." In response to the question, "During sex how important is the girth of the man's penis," 46% said "very important," 46% said "somewhat important," and 8% said "not important." On the basis of the Edward's survey it would appear that girth is more important than length to women.

Blanchard and Levine (1996) interviewed 300 persons but did not describe them or the method of obtaining subjects for their article in Marie Clair magazine.

When Blanchard and Levine asked their interviewees if penis size matters, 77% of the women said yes and 23% said no. In response to the question "Penis size makes up what percentage of your sexual satisfaction," 39% of their subjects said less than 25%, 40% said approximately 50%, 16% said approximately 75%, and 5% said 100%.

Blanchard and Levine asked their female subjects their ideal erect penis size. One percent said 2"-4", 33% said 4"-6", 50% said 6"-8", 8% said over 8", and 8% said size did not matter. It is apparent in the Blanchard and Levine survey that most women preferred men with average or above average but not huge penises.

One of their subjects said, "Huge or tiny is a drag, but almost anything in between is just right."

Blanchard and Levine reported the following comments from women who prefer large penises:

"The bigger the better. For some primal unexplained reason, large penises are a big turn-on."

"People don't want size to matter, but it does. I was with one guy who was small and I wasn't happy about it."

"If his penis is so small it can't hold a condom, or he keeps slipping out; that's a problem. But that also is really rare."

When people speak of penis size they usually talk about the length. However, it is possible that girth is more important to women. When Blanchard and Levine asked women which is more important, 36% said length and 64% said girth. One if the interviewees said:

"Girth. You don't want your cervix tickled, you want the walls of your vagina stimulated."

"Nothing turns me off quicker than a guy with a really skinny penis."

One woman was very emphatic about not wanting an extra large penis:

"I had a boyfriend who was huge. I was in pain every time we had sex, and I got tons of infections. Extra-large is not always excellent."

Hite (1976) provided the following statements from women who experienced pain from too large a penis and/or penetration that is too deep.

"If the man is larger than average, there is some pain-sometimes too much to have orgasm, and I spend all my time trying to keep him from penetrating too deeply."

"I avoid positions that allow his penis to hit my uterus (like being on the bottom with my legs up). In other positions I can avoid his penis hitting my uterus by tightening the muscles in my vagina or by shifting my hips."

"Sometimes it hurts when he gets carried away with deep hard thrusts when he comes. I get a stomach ache, feel battered, and urination becomes painful."

"I'm easily hurt by too deep penetration or too vigorous thrusting, but adjusting my position to limit penetration usually takes care of it."

"Sometimes it burns if my pubic hair is pulled by my being dry, or him being large, or penetration too sudden or deep. It hurts in another way not to come after a long time, with aching and tightness."

Freyer (1998) surveyed a few men for the magazine Glamour about what women think about penis size and provided some interesting comments:

"I've definitely been too large for some women. Penetration can be uncomfortable for me and painful for my partner; I feel really terrible when I see a lover grimace in bed. Lubrication is a problem too, since women tend to dry up faster when you're big. And there are positions I just can't manage because I'll keep hitting against her cervix. Every guy wants to be huge, but at times, it's more of a hazard than a thrill." Larry, 33

"I've heard female friends blab about the penis lengths of guys they've dated and my conclusion is that women may enjoy trading vital statistics, but in the end, technique matters most. In fact, I was just reading an article in a magazine in which women described the best sex they've ever had and not one mentioned the man's equipment. As the saying goes, 'It's not the size of the stick, it's the magic in the wand." Kevin, 30

"I'm only about four or five inches, and I know I've been with women I haven't fully satisfied. They keep grinding against me, like they're hoping I'm going to grow another few inches. I try to please lovers in other ways, with lots of foreplay and hand and tongue stimulation. When the lights are out I can swivel my hips better than Elvis did! But the bottom line is, no relationship that's based on sex will last. You want a woman who cares about what's inside you—not what's dangling outside." Gary, 26

"I say a woman's size is just as important as a man's. I've been lost with big-boned lovers and felt lost inside of them and petite women who were uncomfortably small. The key is for partners to be a good match. Too much in either direction is not good." Tom, 28

"Lots of guys drool over big-breasted women because we're *supposed* to lust after them, and I assume that if women had a choice, many of them would prefer a large man for the same reason. I guess that's always made me a little self-conscious when I'm first with someone, since I'm just average size from what I've seen. Luckily, it's a lot harder for a woman to estimate

Donald I. Templer, Ph.D.

the size of a guy's package before deciding whether or not she's interested." Jeff, 34

PART B: OPINIONS OF GYNECOLOGISTS

Common sense tells us that a larger penis would be more difficult for women who already have penetration or intercourse problems from such conditions as insufficient lubrication, vaginismus (contraction of muscles surrounding vaginal opening so as to prohibit penetration), dysparenuria (painful intercourse), very small vagina, structural abnormalities, and post menopausal vaginal atrophy. Common sense also tells us that if a vagina is very large or very elastic, a small penis provides less stimulation. The following opinions have been given by various gynecologists:

Bahr (1976) stated:

"Sex therapists and gynecologists are far more familiar with female complaints of pain created by large male organs than by expressions of dissatisfaction with inadequate penetration. Frequently, extended oral intercourse is impossible for the woman whose partner has a larger than average phallus. Sexual activity is therefore limited to the more routine genital-to-genital contact and masturbation. And, although apparently no formal study has ever been conducted to prove it, a widely held opinion is that particularly large penises do not attain the degree of rigidity in erection that is achieved by smaller ones. All in all, it is probably the man with the normal size penis rather than the Ringling Brothers extravaganza who is most fortunate."

70

Rosenbaum (1976), Director of Human Sexuality at Albert Einstein College of Medicine, stated:

"However, at each end of the spectrum—the exceptionally large or exceptionally small penis—there may be concrete physical difficulties at times. The too-small penis may not be able to provide enough stimulation and the very large penis may be difficult to accommodate, especially by a not fully stimulated vagina. Both can usually be circumvented by adequate ancillary stimulation of the clitoris or changes in posture. True physical incompatibility is very rare. We tend to focus on length when penis size is discussed. Chances are, however, that the important variable is the diameter. Some women report that a penis with larger diameter is more adept at providing stimulation, presumably by increased traction on the clitoral hood."

Keller (1976), of Cornell Medical College faculty and Sexual Disorder Clinic at Pace University, did not provide the details regarding interviews with 57 sexually active women averaging 4.2 partners in the last two years. We may not be able to make inferences that extend to less (or to more) sexually active women. Nevertheless, her scholarly work is worthy of being quoted:

"But sexually active females who are in a position to assess and assay the effectiveness of male sexual functioning consistently report that men with similar techniques using similar positions during sexual intercourse, but with penises of differing lengths and/or widths, create differing degrees of sexual pleasure.

Donald I. Templer, Ph.D.

They state that the sexual enjoyment has two deter-
minants: real and imagined, physical and fantasized. It is
in direct proportion to penis length for some; it is in direct
proportion to penis width for others; it is in direct proportion to penis length and width for almost all.

"In interviews conducted with 57 sexually active
women, ranging in ages from 17 to 52 averaging 4.2 partners over a period of two years, all but six reported being
more stimulated either by the physical presence of, or
fantasized pleasure of, the bigger penis. With respect to
penis length, women report heightened pleasurable stimulation afforded by the longer penis thrusting against the
cervix. Evidently some women find the stimulation of the
cervix and perhaps the resultant pushing or movement of
the uterus an additional factor in sexual arousal. Pressure
and pushing against and around the cervix is reported by
many women as erotic stimuli which can be felt only in
certain positions (such as female superior) with a partner
having an average size penis. With a long penis these sensations are invariably experienced."

"With respect to penis width, women report heightened pleasurable sensation afforded by the wider penis as
it moves from the introitus into the vagina itself. The
areas of the outer third of the vagina are exquisitely more
sensitive, and many women report extreme pleasure on
being truly filled."

"For years women have been plagued by male fantasies and choice based on breast size. A parallel does
exist: for women, sex does arouse erotic object choice
based on size too. Men with larger penises are sexually

more stimulating to many women, physically and in fantasy."

The bigness or smallness of any penis is to a large extent a function of vaginal size of the woman with whom he is having sex. Although Masters and Johnson assert that genital size is ordinarily of little importance, they did provide case material on a woman with a very large vagina who had insufficient feel of the penis. Masters and Johnson (1966) stated:

"There are occasional women with exceptionally large or small vaginas, just as there are occasional men with an exceptionally large or small penis. The large vagina reacts as an obstetrically traumatized vagina and expands voluntarily far beyond the point of physiologic demand. Only one exceptionally large vagina was identified among the study-subject population of 382 women. The anatomic anomaly rendered immediate accommodation regardless of the size of the artificial penis introduced. A normal-sized penis could be accommodated in this large vagina without an obvious reaction. Therefore, there was little involuntary distention or "tenting" of the vaginal walls. With a twice-normal-sized penis introduced, the large vagina evidenced the involuntary accommodation reaction, expanding and extending in the usual manner. This woman's constant complaint was that during coition the penis seemed lost in the vagina and provided little direct exteroceptive stimulation during thrusting episodes."

Donald I. Templer, Ph.D.

Crenshaw stated on the basis of her experience as a gynecologist:
"Women rarely comment on a man's penis size sponta-
neously. However, when asked, many express a preference for an average-size penis and some for a larger than
average penis. I hear many more comments, however
from women complaining about a larger than average
penis, due to discomfort caused as a result of deep penetration and as a result of particularly large girth. I rarely
hear a woman complain about a man's penis being too
small. Naturally, average to smaller size penises are
unlikely to cause discomfort with intercourse. I occasionally have women who emphatically comment that they
prefer smaller penises and will avoid men who are 'well
endowed.'"

Danoff (1993) stated:
"Certainly, a woman with an exceptionally large vagina
and a man with a very small penis might be sexually
incompatible due to the relative size of their genitals. But
the possibility of a major mismatch is relatively remote.
Lovers, like water, tend to seek their own levels. However,
I do know of such a couple. The woman was nearly a foot
taller than the man. They were hopelessly in love but dissatisfied sexually because, they believed, his penis was
the wrong size for her vagina. But through experimenta-
tion they learned to adjust their positions and angles during intercourse and to vary their sexual practices so that
eventually both were more than content."

Stone and Stone (1952) stated:

"When the vaginal walls are very much relaxed and dis-tended, as, for instance, after difficult childbirths, there may be, it is true, a lack of sufficient contact and some diminution in sexual stimulation and gratification. In modern obstetric practice, however, such relaxations are now being prevented to a considerable extent, or else they are surgically repaired soon after labor. Even if such a condition does exist, a suitable adjustment can still be made. By using her vaginal muscles and learning to tight-en and relax them from time to time during the sexual act, the wife can bring about a much closer contact of the gen-ital organs and increase the sensations both for herself and her husband."

Editor (1992) discussed the matter of pain during inter-course and stated that small vaginal size is not usually the problem but that it can result from genital surgery, radiation therapy, a drug called DES, and menopause. Although large penis size was not mentioned, it is apparent that the largeness or smallness of vaginal size is to some extent a function of penis smallness or largeness. Furthermore, the author did state that deep penetration should be avoided in some condi-tions that produce painful intercourse.

The journal *Medical Aspects of Human Sexuality* asked four experts on human sexuality in the October 1974 issue "What can be done to increase sensation in cases of vaginal stretching?"

Burchell, Hospital Director of Obstetrics and Gynecology, began his comments by saying, "A tight vagina is too often considered the sine qua non for satisfactory coitus." He went on to say:

"Decreased sensation may result from vaginal or cervical infections when there is a discharge. Some discharges tend to be lubricating; cervical infections often cause increased mucus secretion resulting increased lubrication and decreased sensation.

"A practical measure to overcome the complaint of lessened sensation is first to put the problem in perspective and make sure that it is not totally based on a remembered fantasy. Vaginitis and cervicitis causing excess mucus secretion should be ruled out. A gynecologist may not recognize the problem unless the patient is specific. Remember that some couples are overjoyed that extra lubrication decreases sensation and prolongs intromission prior to ejaculation.

"Contraceptive methods may be an additional factor affecting lubrication. Some women have more normal cervical secretions on one birth control pill than another. It may be advisable to change birth control pills with the physician's advice. Jellies are generally less lubricating than creams or foams, and a diaphragm and cream would be less lubricating than creams or foams, and a diaphragm and cream would be less lubricating than cream alone. With respect to mechanical and chemical methods of contraception, a diaphragm and jelly would result in the greatest sensation, and a condom and foam would probably result in the least sensation.

"Some coital positions offer more penile stimulation than others. In general there is less pressure but more penetration when the penis and vagina are on the same axis. Greater pressure and stimulation occur when the axis of the vagina is changed by extension or extreme flexion of the woman's hips. Considering that the upper vagina is distended prior to orgasm, there may be greater penile stimulation if there is only slight penetration so that the glans of the penis remains in the outer third of the vagina. Couples should experiment with different positions to find those which produce the desired sensation."

Moulton, faculty member of William Allen White Institute for Psychiatry, Psychology, and Psychoanalysis, said:

"Another factor which may be over looked is that many older men sustain much less firm erections than they did in their youth. This means that the penis is smaller while the vagina is larger. One way in which the mature woman can help compensate for this discrepancy is to be more active in stimulating her husband rather than playing the role of the young woman who insists on being seduced and pursued. Likewise, the husband may have to spend more time in foreplay since his wife may take longer to become aroused."

Settlage, faculty member of Obstetrics and Gynecology at University of Southern California, said:

"Moreover, as a female gynecologist, I find that as many women complain of vaginal laxity as state that their husbands complain about their condition. The incidence of this type of complaint in response to a routine sexual history is very common whether or not sexual dysfunction exists. Spontaneous volunteering of these complaints should alert the physician to the high probability of sexual relationship difficulties, a lesser probability of pelvic floor damage, or both.

"The gaping introitus, which refers to the introital area and the distal third of the vagina, poses sensory problems for both males and females during intercourse. For the male there may be virtually no gripping or penetration sensation with resultant decrease in friction from coitus. For the female there will be lessened friction and sensation in the introital area. Also, because the penis is not too tightly gripped, indirect stimulation of the labia minora and clitoris is greatly diminished. Improvement in muscle function, allowing greater vulvar stimulation, can be very effective in treating the anorgasmic or hypoesthetic woman who also has poor pubococcygeal muscle tone.

"However, most women with a large introitus and 'vaginal stretching' complaints have demonstrably lax tone of the pubococcygeal muscle rather than obvious separation or damage. Diagnosis of this condition may require specific repeated instruction to appropriately assess contractile ability. Total inability to squeeze the examiner's fingers usually means lack of comprehension of instructions rather than severe nerve or muscle damage. The physician should instruct the patient to squeeze her buttocks together, similar to the squeeze at the end of urination or defecation, and should describe the sensation as similar to lifting up her buttocks and vagina. In addition, adequacy of the anal sphincter reflex usually indicates that the pubococcygeal muscle is neurologically intact.

"Those women who demonstrate poor contractile ability of an intact muscle need to be instructed in Kegel's exercises. These consist of in squeezing the buttocks, anal sphincter, and pubococcygeal muscle as tightly as possible, holding the contraction for 10 seconds, relaxing completely, and then resqueezing in a series of 10 to 20 contractions three or four times a day. I instruct patients to insert their fingers in their vagina and squeeze around them while lying on their back with their knees flexed to determine the strength of the contraction. Once they are able to contract easily, they may use the squatting position for finger-monitored contractions and perform multiple contractions at other times without interrupting their daily routines (as with other isometric exercises).

"A wide variety of instruments have been developed to help exercise the pubococcygeal muscle and to measure the contractile force. Kegel's perineometer and Gynetone operate on this principle. Their advantage is that they come with detailed instructions for performing Kegel's exercises and can be used by scientists to give an objective parameter of increased muscle tone. They are not essential to the exercises, however, and use of the women's own fingers as the object against which to contract has several advantages. She can sensorily appreciate the contracting both pelvically and tactilely."

Semmens, Department of Obstetrics and Obstetrics faculty member of the Medical University of South Carolina, stated:

"Occasionally we see the parous woman whose labia gape and barely cover the vaginal introitus, whose anterior and/or posterior vaginal walls bulge through the opening (cystocele and rectocele) and lack turgor, color, and normal rugal formation. There may even be perineal defects from poorly healed episiotomy scars, especially those of the mesiolateral variety. These findings at vaginal examination are typical of the dysfunctional female, the nonorgasmic female, the female who has lost a desire for sexual relations or simply participates to please her partner. Both partners struggle to improve their relationship, and with repeated failure withdraw from further attempts at coitus. What they fail to realize is that the muscles and fascia of the pelvic diaphragm (pelvic floor) are responsive to exercise and can be brought back to their normal tonic state, once more being capable of supporting the pelvic structures (the uterus and adnexa, bladder, rectum, etc.). Bladder, bowel and sexual functions, as well as a sense of well being, return. Women must be made aware of the effects of prolonged labor, or bearing down to move their bowels, standing for long periods of time, and failing to exercise the perineal muscles."

Chez, Chief of Pregnancy Branch of the National Institute of Health, said:

"Many wives complain of lessened sensation due to vaginal stretching. Most of these women are not recognized by the clinician who does not directly ask the patient about this complaint. I do not usually elicit this information from a patient while obtaining a routine sexual history using open-ended questions. Rather, it requires direct questioning, either in the intake interview or during the pelvic examination when I recognize that an anatomic defect is present.

"Several physical means can be used to increase friction. Direct digital clitoral stimulation by either partner with the couple lying on their side during intercourse can frequently provide increased pleasure for the woman. This is particularly applicable if the vaginal relaxation is such that penile thrust does not result in movement of the labia minora and perineum with resultant absence of clitoral stimulation. Either partner can direct the erect penis against a particular area of the vagina. Angling the penis in such a way that the glans is directed against the anterior vaginal wall is frequently helpful. Insertion from behind can accomplish this as well. The woman can take one or both of her hands and stretch the skin at the base of the penis against the man's pubis, thereby heightening sensation on the stretched glans. Or she can place her hands on the shaft of the penis near its base and by varying pressure simulate vaginal barrel friction. Saliva or vaginal secretions will lubricate the hands. Similarly, pressure along the later aspects of the labia against the shaft of the penis can enhance sensation for both partners.

"The role of vaginoplasty and specifically an operative buildup of the perineal body must be considered. Some physicians advocate this surgical approach, and there is no reason to doubt its effectiveness. Certainly one of the results of vaginal surgery for urinary incontinence is a tightening of the vaginal barrel. However, physicians seem reluctant to do vaginal surgery primarily to increase sexual pleasure."

Danoff (1993) said:

"A much more common complaint is that a lover's penis is too big. Intercourse can be painful for a woman whose vagina can't accommodate a large penis. I have actually had women ask me to surgically reduce the size of their husband's penis. There is no such procedure—just as there is no procedure to make them bigger.

"One source of pain, however, is biologically determined: his penis is too big. As I've already mentioned, I have had many more requests to make a husband's penis shorter or thinner than to make it longer or wider. Unfortunately, there is no medical solution. The answer is to adjust the angle of penetration and the depth of insertion until you find a combination that is both satisfying and comfortable. Remember also: there is no rule that says a penis has to penetrate to its full length."

Lanson (1975) maintained that ordinarily a man's penis is not important with respect to satisfying a woman. Nevertheless, she did say there are exceptions:

"Where the penis is so large as to cause actual discomfort despite adequate lubrication and a normally accommodating vagina; and when the penis is so abnormally small that effective coital contact cannot be maintained."

Lanson went on to answer two relevant questions:

"Can vaginal size affect a woman's enjoyment of intercourse?"

Although there are a few women who do have an exceptionally small or large vagina, they are just that - exceptions. Since the vaginal walls normally lie against each other, most healthy average vaginas effectively ensheathe the penis during intercourse. This close contact between the penis and the vaginal walls enhances physical enjoyment for both partners. With continued stimulation and arousal, the normal vagina will dilate and expand to accommodate deep thrusting by almost any size penis.

"However, difficulties during first intercourse can be encountered if the woman has too snug a vaginal opening. This is occasionally seen in women who have never used tampons or have never engaged in sexual play wherein the vaginal opening was dilated manually. For such women, pain at the vaginal opening during penetration or, less commonly, complete inability to permit penile entry can definitely be a detriment to sexual enjoyment. Fortunately, however, a hymen rarely offers much resistance to firm but gentle stretching. In fact, if the woman is sufficiently aroused and lubricated, penile penetration even the first time can frequently be accomplished with little difficulty. The idea that all first intercourse must be accompanied by pain and obvious hymenal bleeding just isn't so.

"The opposite problem, a too relaxed vagina, is not only a common complaint of many women but may also be a source of sexual dissatisfaction for some. Most

women who express concern about a too relaxed or overly stretched vagina are usually in their late thirties or for-
ties and have had at least two children. Even with the best
obstetrical care, the unavoidable strain and stress of child-
bearing can weaken and disrupt the normally firm muscle
and connective tissue supports of the vaginal walls and
introitus. The vaginas of these women tend to become
wider, shorter, and less capable of making tight contact
with the penetrating penis. Women who have this problem
will notice that the penis no longer seems to fill the vagina. And their partners will complain that their organ feels
lost inside. For some couples, this relative disproportion
between penis and vagina, although a source of decreased
sensory awareness, does not detract from their enjoyment
of the sexual act.

"For other women, a too relaxed *vaginal opening* may
also interfere with clitoral stimulation during coitus. In
these instances effective *indirect* clitoral stimulation,
which normally occurs when downward traction is exert-
ed on the labia and clitoral hood during active penile
thrusting, is greatly impaired."

**Can anything be done for the vagina and introitus that
seem too large?**

"Very definitely. Where an overly stretched vagina
seems to be interfering with the full enjoyment of sexual
intercourse, a change in coital position may be helpful.
Since the object is to tighten the vaginal canal as well as
the vaginal opening, some women find that bringing their
legs together once the penis has been introduced allows

for closer contact. This maneuver is easily accomplished if the woman lies on her back while the male partner, on top, places his legs outside of hers.

"If a too relaxed vaginal opening prevents adequate indirect clitoral stimulation during coitus, the woman-on-top position or the side-by-side position can help resolve the problem. In either of these positions, direct clitoral stimulation can occur during deep penile penetration.

"For women, however, whose main concern is a too wide or relaxed vaginal canal, a more satisfactory solution (other than changing coital position) would be the firming and strengthening of certain pelvic muscles essential for the maintenance of normal vaginal tone. Exercising the pubococcygeus (Kegel's exercises) can significantly improve a too relaxed vagina.

"If vaginal relaxation or stretching has progressed beyond the help of corrective exercises, vaginal plastic surgery is an effective procedure for restoring the vagina to more normal dimensions. Although most vaginal plastic procedures are done to alleviate the symptoms associated with the prolapse of pelvic organs, such as the bladder, more and more gynecologists are accepting the idea that tightening the vaginal canal and introitus when specifically requested to enhance sexual enjoyment is a warranted procedure."

PART C: MISCELLANEOUS MATERIAL

At least in the past, there were a number of reported cases in India in which little girls suffered injuries, sometimes very seriously so, from the penis of an adult male to whom they were married. We Americans are justified in criticizing such practices in cultures that are different from ours. We should, however, bear in mind the fact that the same sort of injuries take place in the United States when prepubescent girls are raped or molested.

Calderood (1987) estimated that anal sex occurs in 50% of married or cohabitating heterosexual couples:

"Most often, the man who prefers anal intercourse does so because the partner's anal sphincter is tighter and provides more friction for the penis than her vagina. Exercises to return good muscle tone to the vagina can restore both partner's interest in and satisfaction for this more traditional form of intercourse."

I wish to point out that anal sex does contain risks of disease and injury. Travis and Sadd (1977) said that some physicians maintain that such problems are more common if the penis is large.

Size of penis may sometimes be a factor in condom failure. In a survey of 127 female prostitutes and 91 clients in the Netherlands (de Graaf, Vanwesenbeeck, van Zessen, Straver, & Visser, 1993), 62% of the prostitutes and 9% of the clients attributed condom slipping off before ejaculation to the penis being too small. Twenty-six percent of the prostitutes but none of the clients attributed condom breakage to a penis being too large. Seven percent of the prostitutes expressed a need for smaller (more slender) condoms, 11% larger (broader) condoms, and 18% both larger and smaller condoms. Three percent of the clients expressed the need for more slender and 10% broader condoms. Chapter 4 on ethnic differences indicated that African American men are more likely to have condom breakage.

Research of Smith, Jolley, Hocking, Benton, and Gerofi (1998) found that men with large penises were more likely to experience condom breakage, and men with small penises were more likely to have the condom slip off. Apparently penis girth is a more important factor than condom length. Smith et al. recommended that condom manufacturers market a greater range of condom sizes.

Donald I. Templer, Ph.D.

PRACTICAL IMPLICATIONS

For the vast majority of couples size incompatibility is not a problem. For the minority of couples for which it is a problem, it can be effectively resolved. Patience, time, common sense, and using optimal techniques will often take care of the matter. If a woman has had little or no previous sexual intercourse, the initial difficulty in intromission (insertion of the penis) and soreness after intercourse will decrease as her vagina becomes less "tight" as more intercourse takes place. If a man's penis is thicker than ideal for his partner's vagina, inserting the penis slowly and employing a lubricant often solves the problem. There are times when the apparent problem of excessive girth is really a problem of not waiting for sufficient female arousal and associated increased vaginal lubrication. If a man's penis is too long for the woman's vagina, the couple should use a position in which less penetration takes place or simply have the man not penetrate to the extent that discomfort occurs. This ordinarily does not decrease the man's pleasure.

If a man's penis is too thin for a snug fit in the woman's vagina, artificial lubrication should ordinarily not be employed. In fact, the couple may consider drying the vagina with a handkerchief if there is excessive natural vaginal lubrication. The insufficient snugness often results not from size incompatibility but from excessive vaginal lubrication. If a woman's vagina has increased in girth and/or lost tone from childbirth, Kegel exercise may be employed. If a man's penis is too short for a woman, the couple can employ positions that involve maximum penetration.

It is possible for a man's penis to be less than ideal and more than ideal in length in the same night of love making. It may also be too thick and too thin in that same night, depending upon the positions employed, degree of sexual arousal, the amount of naturally secreted vaginal lubrication, and the possible use of artificial lubrication. And, there may be changes in ideal over a long term relationship that occur as a function of such factors as sexual experience, childbirth, decrease in vaginal size and lubrication after menopause, hormonal changes, surgery, and other health problems.

One possible solution to less-than-preferred girth and less-than-preferred length is that of surgery and other techniques to increase penile girth and/or length as described in Chapter 8, "Methods Used to Increase Penis Size." As stated in that chapter, there appears to be a paucity of well controlled research to determine the effectiveness and safety of these methods. I would neither strongly encourage nor strongly discourage use of these methods.

The various sexual intercourse positions have advantages and disadvantages in regard to genital size compatibility and to degree and type of sexual stimulation desired. The most commonly used in the United States is the so-called "missionary position," with the woman lying on her back with her legs bent and spread apart and the man on top and facing her. This is a position in which degree of penetration is controlled primarily by the man, and which permits rather deep penetration. If a man has a long penis relative to the length of the woman's vagina, and if he becomes "carried away" at the approach of ejaculation, the woman may experience discomfort. If the woman places her legs on his shoulders, even deeper penetration is possible. If she places her legs inside his legs, there will be less penetration, but greater vaginal "tightness." If she grasps his body with her legs, there will be greater tightness. In general, positions that involve placing the woman's legs closer together narrow the vagina and positions that place her legs further apart expand the vagina. Rear entry positions, which usually involve both partners kneeling or the man and woman lying on their sides, are positions that bring about shallow penetration and vaginal narrowness. The woman can have a great deal of control of degree of penetration if she sits on a man's lap while he sits on a firm chair, or if he lies on his back and she straddles him. These positions probably permit the greatest degree of penetration. On the other hand, the woman could choose shallow penetration if that's what she prefers. In the side-to-side position, in which the man and woman are facing each other and he has a leg between her legs, penetration is quite shallow.

If a woman has a definite strong preference for men with very large or very small penises her preference should be regarded as a legitimate one. She should not be told that she is mentally disturbed and should seek psychotherapy. She should instead seek a sex partner with the penis dimensions that she prefers. Such decisions should be made in the context of her overall values and circumstances. I would not encourage either a man or a woman to break up a happy marriage and make children miserable merely to obtain a little more sexual pleasure. This chapter ends with Barach's (1984) good description of the Kegel exercises.

THE KEGEL EXERCISES

In the mid-1900s, Dr. Kegel developed a series of exercises to help women who suffered from urinary incontinence, i.e., they would inadvertently expel small amounts of urine if they coughed, sneezed, or had an orgasm. The exercises consisted of strengthening the pubococcygeal (PC) muscle, the muscle that, when squeezed, stops the flow of urine. The PC muscle turns out to be the same muscle that forms the orgasmic platform and, along with other pelvic muscles, contracts with orgasm. Consequently, when Kegel questioned women about their response to his exercises, they replied that not only was their ability to retain urine better after practicing the exercises, but they were experiencing more sexual sensations during intercourse as well. Kegel exercises are also recommended both before and after childbirth as a way of toning and strengthening the vagina. Postmenopausal women who use Kegel exercises find that they help to maintain lubrication by increasing bloodflow to the vaginal area and reduce the need for estrogen creams.

First, to locate the PC muscle, urinate with your legs apart; the muscle you squeeze to stop the flow of urine is the PC muscle. Practice stopping the flow of urine a few times in order to become familiar with the muscle. Then, lie down and put your finger in the opening of your vagina and contract the PC muscle. See if you can feel the contraction around your finger while taking care not to move your thighs, stomach, buttocks, or any other muscles in the pelvic region.

After practicing the following exercises for about six weeks, see if you notice any difference in the strength of your PC muscle when you put your finger in your vagina and squeeze.

91

Donald I. Templer, Ph.D.

THE SQUEEZE-RELEASE EXERCISE

The first Kegel exercise consists of squeezing the PC muscle for three seconds, relaxing the muscle for three seconds, and squeezing it again. It may be difficult, at first, to contract the muscle for a full three seconds. If this is the case, contract for one or two seconds at first and build up the time as the muscle gets stronger. Carry out a series of ten squeezes at three different times during the day.

THE FLUTTER EXERCISE

The second exercise is much like the first except that instead of holding the squeeze for three seconds, the objective is to squeeze the muscle, relax it, squeeze again, and release as quickly as possible. Again, complete a series of ten squeezes and releases at three different times during the day.

When you first start doing this exercise, it may feel like a tongue twister; you may not be able to tell if you are contracting or releasing and for a while it may feel all muddled together. However, begin slowly and with practice you will gradually be able to do the Flutter more rapidly.

THE ELEVATOR EXERCISE

The third exercise consists of exercising the entire length of the vagina. Imagine that your vagina is an elevator shaft and the elevator is at the opening to the vagina. Rather than squeezing, contract the muscles as you imagine yourself slowly pulling the elevator upward along the vaginal canal,

92

beginning at the opening and ending at the uterus. After the three or four seconds it takes to go the entire length of the vagina, slowly relax the muscles as if you were lowering the elevator to the ground floor, and then begin again at the vaginal opening. Do three series of ten contractions daily. This exercise is good for strengthening the uterine muscles as well as the PC muscle.

The advantage of these first three Kegel exercises is that you can do them anywhere and at any time and no one can tell you're doing them. Practice when you stop the car for a red light or in the morning when you wake up. Or do them when you answer the telephone at home or at work, or when you are lying down to rest. The muscles surrounding your anus may move during these exercises, but if you find you are moving your thigh muscles, your stomach muscles, or your buttocks, you are probably squeezing the wrong muscles.

THE BEARING-DOWN EXERCISE

The fourth exercise is more apparent to the observer, so you might want to practice it in privacy. It consists of bearing down as during a bowel movement, but with the emphasis more on the vagina than the anal area. Imagine there is a tampon deep inside your vagina and bear down as if you were pushing it out. The bearing down should be held for three or four seconds as with the Elevator Exercise.

All four exercises should be practiced ten times each at three different times during the day in the beginning. As you progress with the Kegel exercises, slowly increase the number of repetitions in each series until you are able to do twenty of each exercise in succession. You can do them as frequently during the day as you can find time, but consider three times daily a minimum.

Some women hesitate to practice the Kegel exercises because they feel sexually aroused by contracting the PC muscle. While this can be disconcerting, it is a perfectly normal reaction. The muscle tension created by the exercises causes blood to flow to the pelvic region which is the same physiological process that occurs with sexual stimulation. So, if this happens to you, don't worry about it - just enjoy it. Other women discontinue practicing the Kegel exercises because they find the exercises fatiguing. If this is true for you, you are probably using muscles in your abdomen, buttocks, or thighs rather than exercising the PC muscle by itself. In this case, begin again by stopping the flow of urine without squeezing the muscles in the abdomen, buttocks, or thigh areas to isolate the correct muscle.

If you are carrying out the exercise correctly, but you initially notice some discomfort or tightness in the pelvic region, reduce the number of daily contractions, but do not abandon the exercises. Like any muscle that is being exercised for the first time, it may feel a little still initially. However, it is quite important to keep this muscle, like others in your body, in tone. The Kegel exercises should become as much of a habit as brushing your teeth, and, like brushing your teeth, should be continued for the rest of your life.

CHAPTER 7

PENIS SIZE IN FANTASIES OF WOMEN

There have been at least five interview-based investigations on the sexual fantasy life of women. These investigations are contained in the books *My Secret Garden* by Nancy Friday (1973), *In the Garden of Desire* by Wendy Maltz and Suzie Boss (1997), Rosemary Santini's (1976) *The Secret of Fire*, Karen Shanor's (1977) *A Study of the Sexual Fantasies of Contemporary Women*, and Nancy Friday's (1991) *Women on Top*. These investigations seem like credible ones. The authors, however, did not obtain a random or representative sample of American women. Therefore, we cannot be certain about what percentage of women have sexual fantasies that involve penis size. What we do know is that in the total of 63 fantasies involving penis size in these books, the penises are described as large in 61 (97%) of the fantasies. Words such as "big," "huge," "large," "long," "eight inches," "ten inches," "thick," and "fat" are often used. Although the ethnicity of the men possessing the penises is ordinarily not reported, when the men are described as black, the penises are always described as exceptionally large.

Table 7.1 contains the description of penis size, the other physical characteristics of the men (or boys or animals), and place and circumstances of the fantasy event, in each of the 63 fantasies. In Nancy Friday's (1991) Women on Top fantasies numbers 14a and 14b are of two distinct fantasies of one women. And, fantasy 20a and 20b also are two distinct fantasies of one woman. The other 59 fantasies are of 59 different women.

Table 7.1 Description of penis size in 63 fantasies of women

Author & book Title	Fantasy #	Description of penis size	Other characteristics of man	Place & circumstances (if specified)
Rosemary Santini (1976)	1	"large penis"	"Black boys" who were Mugging commuters	forcefully sodomized (penis in rectum) in subway station
Wendy Maltz & Suzie Boss (1997) In the Garden of Desire	1	"large penis"	handsome, tanned, blond lean, muscular, tight buttocks	sexual intercourse with her in room at ski lodge
Karen Shanor (1977) A Study of Sexual Fantasies in Contemporary Women	1	"large penis"	black man, body in good shape and shiny	sexual intercourse with her
	2	"giant and red"	bull was huge and strong and persistent	bull copulating with cows
	3	"huge erections"	"horney guys" one after the other.	sexual intercourse with her,
	4	"big (penis)"	handsome man	having intercourse with her at wild party
	5	"giant penis"	tall dark man	rapes her in her house
	6	"2 inches in diameter"	men	having sexual intercourse with her
	7	"oversized penis"	really beautiful guy	having sexual intercourse with her

97

Table 7.1 (con't)

Author & book Title	Fantasy #	Description of penis size	Other characteristics of man	Place & circumstances (if specified)
Nancy Friday (1991) *Women on Top*	1	"big hard (sexual intercourse) tool"	a professional, large-framed, somewhat of a pot belly, not Romeo type, not flirty or aggressive with women, does not radiate sex appeal (a person she actually knows)	having intercourse and a variety of sexual activities with her
	2	"naturally long (penis)"	has a large scrotum	having sexual intercourse with her - a previous lover
	3	"huge," "12 inches long," "well endowed"	her favorite actor masculine, adored by women, lovely build	having sexual intercourse with her in his hotel room
Nancy Friday's (1991) *Women on Top*	4	"big and fat"	broad shouldered, arms long-muscled	
	5	all "well-endowed"	very nice builds, some blond, some brunettes, some Italian, a couple of black men	15 different male housekeepers. Sexual intercourse with different one every night in her home
	6	"large (penis)"	minister at church	intercourse with her in abandoned building

98

Table 7.1 (con't)

Author & book Title	Fantasy #	Description of penis size	Other characteristics of man	Place & circumstances (if specified)
	7	"big"	small and very attractive	sexual intercourse with her in abandoned building
	8	"big (penis)"	her new boss	having sexual intercourse in chair in his office
	9	"huge"	good looking black man	having sexual intercourse with her in bedroom
	10	"not long but thick"	handsome man, slightly sweaty and dirty from labor, bulging muscles, hands big and strong	intercourse with her in bedroom
	11	"nine inches"	her first lover	group sex in very luxurious hotel room
	12	"well endowed"	men	group of men raping her in her bedroom
	13	"big thick (penis)"	man with large hands	king size bed
	14a	"10 inches long," "I can barely get fingers around it"	man	anal intercourse with her on bed

99

Table 7.1 (con't)

Author & book Title	Fantasy #	Description of penis size	Other characteristics of man	Place & circumstances (if specified)
Nancy Friday's (1991) *Women on Top*	14b	"(penis) is monstrously large"	some man professor or distant relative or vampire	sexual intercourse with her in her bedroom
	15	"enormous penis"	big man and little effeminate man	sex party at her house. big man inserts penis into anus of little man
	16	"14 inches long and real thick" "12 inches long"	Italian man (good looking and husky)	in her bedroom Italian man has anal intercourse with her and black man inserts penis into her mouth
	17	"huge (penis)"	muscular man	sexual intercourse with her in her house
	18	"8 3/4 inches"	boyfriend - friend	his penis sucked by her in group sex scene
	19	"huge (penis)"	black and muscular	group sex in the Caribbean. One man has anal sex with her as another man has vaginal sex with her. She does not specify which has "huge (penis)"
	20a	"huge (penis)"	homosexual friend	man has anal intercourse with other men and with women

Table 7.1 (con't)

Author & book Title	Fantasy #	Description of penis size	Other characteristics of man	Place & circumstances (if specified)
	20b	"huge penis"	big brawny hunter	he and she independently masturbate and he then inserts gun into her vagina
	21	"huge (penis)" "10 inches long and 8 inches around"	fantasizes herself as man with huge penis	masturbates with her penis
Nancy Friday's (1991) *Women on Top*	22	"big (penis)"	stranger	while in bondage, and after another woman performs oral sex upon her, the man has sexual intercourse with her
	23a	"hairless little erections"	3 little boys 12, 13, maybe 14 ["a beautiful young Adonis," the one she has sex with]	"tip of his perfect maleness begins beating away on my stiff little clitoris"
	23b	"huge pink wet (penis)"	large dog	has sexual intercourse with her
	24	"12 inches long and 2 inches in diameter" "huge (penis)"	a male gorilla	has sexual intercourse with her for scientific experiment movie
	25	"huge dog (penis)"	German Shepherd	has anal intercourse with her in bedroom
	26	"enormous (penis)"	biker	has her suck his penis while other bikers watch

Table 7.1 (con't)

Author & book Title	Fantasy #	Description of penis size	Other characteristics of man	Place & circumstances (if specified)
Nancy Friday's (1973) *My Secret Garden*	1	"big and stiff" "massive (penis)"	big black man	forced to suck mans penis in big house
	2	"big bulge" "I didn't think it so big"	younger man	stroked penis of stepson in bedroom. Was going to have intercourse but he ejaculated prematurely
	3	"enormous penis"	a bull	fantasizes bull's penis in her vagina while she has sexual intercourse with husband
	4	"nine and twelve inches"	men	her being raped by 3 or 4 men with each man having a larger penis than previous man
Nancy Friday's (1973) *My Secret Garden*	5	"long animal maleness"	young male dog	exual intercourse with her while he is being whipped by another man
	6	"enormous (penis)"	dark and good lookings	sexual intercourse with her while she is in stirrups of gynecological table and being watched by thousands of men
	7	"giant erection" "enormous erection"	man	
	8	"well endowed"	very handsome, dark hair, muscular	her being raped by men or group of men
	9	"enormous erect penis"	man	sexual intercourse

Table 7.1 (con't)

Author & book Title	Fantasy #	Description of penis size	Other characteristics of man	Place & circumstances (if specified)
	10	"big erection"	man	being spanked by man as she looks at his erect penis
	11	"immensely huge penis"	nothing or no one on end of penis	brutal men break her bones and rip her body apart
	12	"enormous erection"	man	sucking man's penis after he spanks her
	13	"long and slim"	dark hair on head	sexual intercourse
	14	"exceptionally large"	man	woman or nurse who brings patient in hospital to climax with her hand
	15	"huge (erection)"		sexual intercourse with dog
	16	"massive (penis)"	donkey	forced by other people to have sexual intercourse with donkey
	17	"so big"	very handsome Harry Belafonte-type black man	urinating on her
	18	"the size of his genitalia"	man	watching him masturbating
Nancy Friday's (1973) "My Secret Garden"	19	"broad and stiff" "big (penis)"	man	looking at man's penis
	20	"larger penis" than husband's	man	sexual intercourse

Donald I. Templer, Ph.D.

Table 7.1 (con't)

Author & book Title	Fantasy #	Description of penis size	Other characteristics of man	Place & circumstances (if specified)
	21	"small delicate looking penis"	statue of Greek God Hermes	sexual intercourse with statue of Hermes
	22	"large penis"	dark-skinned Italian man	sexual intercourse
	23	"enormous (penis)" "giant (penis)" shiny	Black man, really black covered with sweat, almost	she puts Tampax in his rectum
	24	"huge penis"		sexual intercourse
	25	"in excess of what I had imagined"	newsboy, fantasizes "young boys"	sexual intercourse in her home
	26	"huge penis" (her husband has small penis)	abnormally big man	sexual intercourse

104

IS SIZE IMPORTANT?

Of the total of 63 fantasies that mention penis size and are described in these five books, only two specify the penises as small, and in both of these the fantazied sex objects are atypical ones. One woman described having sex with a statue of the Greek God Hermes who has a "small, delicate-looking penis." Another woman described having sex with one of three prepubescent boys who had "hairless little (erections)." It should also be noted that no penile penetration was described in this fantasy. The woman said that "the tip of his perfect maleness began beating away on my stiff little (clitoris)." An additional way that her fantasy life is apparently atypical is that in her other fantasy her lover was a dog!

Six of the 63 fantasies described males that were neither men nor boys. They were animals - three dogs, a bull, a donkey, and a gorilla. The woman who fantasized the gorilla with a "huge (penis)," "12 inches long and 2 inches in diameter," probably did not know that gorillas have very small penises. The human male has the largest penis of any primate.

Donald I. Templer, Ph.D.

PRACTICAL IMPLICATIONS

It is quite apparent that when women specify the size of penises in their fantasies, the penises are almost always large. Some of these fantasies involve penises that are more than large. They are huge! We cannot automatically assume that all of these women would want such large penises in their actual sex lives. Although it is fairly common for women to fantasize about physically coerced sex, it is the most unusual woman who wants to be raped.

May I suggest that penis and penis size have three roles in the sex lives of women. One is the stimulation provided by the penis in sexual intercourse. The second is the visual appeal. This is comparable to the visual appeal of breasts to men. Some men like to look at large breasts. Some men prefer medium size breasts, and some men prefer small breasts. On the basis of casual conversation of men, it would appear that most men prefer large breasts. Breasts, however, play very little role in actual sexual intercourse. A third function of the penis is that for some women it is the ultimate symbol of masculinity. The large penis is to masculinity as Cadillacs and caviar and fur coats and country clubs are to wealth. A nice thing about fantasies is that they contain no limits. Their only constrictions are the limitations of our imagination. The man with the huge penis may be, at least to some women, the symbol of all the sexual pleasure and attainment a woman can have.

CHAPTER 8

METHODS USED TO INCREASE PENIS SIZE

In this chapter I merely describe the methods of increasing penis size and what success the advocates report. I do not provide any opinion about whether or not these methods are actually effective. I also do not provide any opinion about their safety. Nevertheless, there are risks in all surgical procedures. One should obtain medical opinion about the safety of surgical and non surgical methods. Also, I am not a clergyman or theologian and therefore have no statements on relevant moral issues. Nevertheless, a number of religions regard masturbation as sinful; and there may be an element of masturbation in some of these methods.

Donald I. Templer, Ph.D.

VACUUM PUMP

The vacuum pump is sold in many adult shops and is advertised in magazines and over the radio. It is said to increase both length and girth, and it is probably the method that is used the most by American men. Those devices that are electrically powered are said by their sellers to be more effective, but are also more expensive. Both sort of pumps operate upon simple laws of physics. The penis, often when already in an erect or semi-erect state, is placed in a transparent cylinder, and when a vacuum is produced in the cylinder, the penis increases in size as more blood flows into the penis to fill the vacuum. There seems to be a general consensus of opinion that the penis enlarges while in the cylinder but that there is a loss of most of this gain over a period of hours. Some authorities claim that one session is enough to produce some permanent increase. Nevertheless, most authorities maintain that the use of the vacuum pump is like body building insofar as it should be carried out for at least a couple of times a week and that one should persevere in such activity for over a year to obtain maximum results. The blood vessels of the penis are said to enlarge over the period of the enlargement program. The enlargement of the penis in some persons is said to be as much as 2" in length, with comparable increase in girth. The increase is manifested in both the flaccid and erect state. Most of the authorities, however, do not claim extremely big gains. It is exceedingly unlikely that a man with a 4" long penis can transform it to a 7" one. It is said that some men also use it as a method of masturbation and that ejaculation can occur. It is claimed that the vacuum pump use does not lead to serious penile injuries, but sessions that are too long and vigorous can produce very small hemorrhages of capillaries on the surface of the penis. These are said to disappear within a few days or so. Also, the penis is said to sometimes take on a blue color, and the authorities maintain that one should wait until normal color appears before the resumption of pumping.

Does the vacuum pump work? Those who sell them say they do. There are apparently enthusiastic testimonials that they are effective. There are before and after pictures that seem to indicate they are effective. I, however, do not know of any well-controlled, scientific studies reported in professional journals that document the efficacy of these methods.

Vacuum constrict devices are also used to induce erection in impotent men. The articles in urological and other professional journals seem to indicate that they are effective for the majority of men who use them. It could be viewed as almost surprising that the physicians who write about the use of vacuum devices for impotency say virtually nothing about whether or not there is increase in size in what might be thought of as a "bonus" of this treatment. Cookson and Nadig (1993), however, did report that 96% of their patients were pleased with the length and circumference of their induced erections. These authors went on to say that the vacuum constriction device produces an erection of greater diameter than in an ordinary erection because of the large amount of blood that is trapped in the penis. These authors did not, however, state whether or not any of this increase is long lasting or permanent. Even some persons who dispute the claims that vacuum devices produce permanent changes acknowledge that there is increase during use and for several hours later.

WEIGHT HANGING

It has been claimed by various persons that hanging a weight from the penis serves to make it larger, at least in length and at least in the flaccid state. It is claimed that this stretches the suspensory ligament. (In the *Surgery* subsection of this chapter the role of this ligament is discussed). Essentially a weight is suspended from the penis in devices that vary from home-made and very unsophisticated to more sophisticated commercial apparatus. One limitation is that these devices are more operational when walking or standing than when seated or lying down. Another limitation is the possibility that others will be able to ascertain the location and movement of the weight through the pants.

WARM WATER

It has been claimed that the placing of the penis in warm water serves to obtain more than temporary enlargement. Also, there is a device on the commercial market that is called an "aqualator" and provides the penis with flowing warm water.

MANUAL METHODS

It is claimed that pulling and stretching the penis a number of times a day brings about enlargement. Such claims are also made for "milking," which consists of squeezing the penis from the top of the shaft downward to the glans. I have heard from more than one person who has worked for institutions for the retarded that the retarded men tend to have large penises. This may or may not be correct. If it is correct it may or may not be related to the fact that quite a few severely retarded men spend a number of hours a day masturbating.

STRETCH STRAP

There are devices on the commercial market that have one end strapped to the penis, the other end to the lower thigh, stretching the penis while connected to both ends. This would appear to have the same sort of effect as hanging a weight from the penis.

RINGS

A ring of plastic, rubber, or metal may be placed around the base of the flaccid penis. Some persons maintain that this is less for enlargement than for maintaining the flaccid penis at maximum flaccid size for whatever reasons one would want to do such, e.g., for maximizing the bulge in one's pants. Probably the main use of the ring is to maintain maximum erection over a longer period of time in sexual intercourse. There is some danger of too small a ring hurting the penis and not being easily removed while the penis is erect.

SURGERY

There are two principal types of surgery to increase penis size. One consists of placing fat from another part of the body into the penis to increase its girth. The other consists of cutting the suspensory ligament to increase penile length. The second was apparently first used in a boy who had most of his penis bitten off by a pig (Hellstrom, 1997).

In the former type of enlargement fat is transferred from another part of the body, such as the abdomen or pubic area or buttocks, to beneath the skin around the penis. Because the glans (head) of the penis has a different structure than the shaft, fat is not inserted into the glans. Most authorities maintain that, in general, the various enlargement techniques are less effective for increasing the size of the glans than the shaft. Surgical girth enlargement is not an extremely minor surgical procedure. And, this and the other surgical procedures are definitely more expensive than the non surgical methods of attempted enlargement. All surgery involves some risk.

To comprehend the suspensory ligament surgery one must understand a couple of facts about the anatomy of the penis. First of all, the penis actually extends 3" inches or so into the body. Secondly, the penis has somewhat of an upward orientation before leaving the body and is held up by a ligament. Thus, if we consider the entire penis, both outside and inside the body, the penis is curved upward before leaving the body and downward after leaving the body. If the suspensory ligament is cut one would expect a straightening of the penis so that it "hangs" lower in the flaccid state. Many authorities maintain that lengthening is more impressive in the flaccid than in the erect state. Some authorities maintain that there is little or no lengthening in the flaccid state. Therefore, this surgery may be more beneficial for showing off in the locker room or nude beach than for bedroom activity.

In 1994, the American Urological Association issued a statement that fat injection and the incision of the suspensory ligament have neither been demonstrated to be safe nor effective procedures. A cosmetic surgeon was convicted of manslaughter because his patient bled to death after the surgery. Another surgeon had his license removed because over 40 of his patients maintained they suffered from ill effects. The cutting of the suspensory ligament is said to at least in some patients result in scarring, decreased ability to have an erection, and actual decrease in penis length. The fat insertion to make the penis thicker may make one's erect penis less hard.

SILICONE INJECTIONS

Christ and Askew (1982) reported on a 42 year old man who received an implant 14 years earlier for the purpose of size augmentation. The results had been satisfactory for the first 11 years. Two years prior to his hospital admission his penis began to increase greatly in size to the point that it became too massive for penetration. Also, he became unable to obtain an erection. Two surgeries were required to remove the abnormal masses. The impotence, however, was permanent, and the patient had to have a penile prosthesis inserted. (These prosthetic devices have limited value and the seemingly erect penis is not as erect as in a normal erect state.)

Christ and Agnew reviewed 4 previous cases of silicone injection reported in the literature. Datta and Kerm (1973) reported on a 45-year-old man who received a silicone injection a year before for impotence. There was no improvement in the problem, but there was deformity and painful erection. Arthaud (1973) reported on a 51-year-old patient who received treatment and a silicone implant 4 years earlier for impotence. The impotence was not improved and a tender mass resulted. Lighterman (1976) reported on 2 cases. One was that of a 38-year-old man who had the implant 7 years earlier for size augmentation. The results were satisfactory and with the bonus of a slight decrease in sensation, preventing premature ejaculation. The other case was that of a 49-year-old man who had the silicone implant 7 years earlier for size augmentation. The results were satisfactory for 3 years until migration of silicone produced hardness and enlargement, preventing penetration.

It appears that silicone injection can be a very dangerous procedure with more risks than benefits. On the basis of these case reports it appears that at least some of these silicone injections were done illegally by persons who don't have medical degrees.

PETROLEUM JELLY ("VASELINE") INJECTION

Douglas (1973) reported the case of a 41-year-old man who 3 years before awoke from a drunken stupor to find his penis swollen and painful. He was informed that his companion injected his penis with Vaseline in an attempt to make it larger. Surgical procedures for the chronically inflamed penis included the removal of dead and fibrous tissue and a skin graft. On the basis of this case, it would not appear that Vaseline injection is a good idea.

Does frequency of use affect the size?

It is common knowledge that not using muscles causes muscular atrophy. One might wonder if disuse of the penis for sex can result in atrophy. In their textbooks on human sexuality Byrne and Byrne (1977) stated that "Sexually active persons are believed to have less size decrease due to the atrophy of aging than those less active. In this way regular sexual indulgence helps prevent loss of size." Byrne and Byrne, however, did not give the research or clinical basis for their assertion.

Getzoff (1972) answered the following question from another doctor: "Is it possible for an impotent man's penis to shrink? One such patient said this is happening and my observations do not allow me to dismiss this as an unfounded expression of anxiety."

Getzoff stated:

"This question implies that actual measurements of the patient's penis were made before the onset of impotence and for a reasonable period of time following the occurrence of this condition. Unfortunately, no mention is made of the etiology of the patient's problem. 'Atrophy of disuse' of the permanent flaccid penis is occasionally mentioned by impotent men, but I have never found this complaint to be confirmed by the patient's wife. Scant attention is given this situation in the urological literature."

Adelson (1976) stated, "Factually, masturbation, whether frequent or not, does not alter the size or rate of growth of the penis." In Adelson's brief note in a correspondence section of a journal, he apparently did not have sufficient space to say how he formed his opinion.

A number of studies have demonstrated that male rats allowed to have sex with female rats achieved greater penis size than rats not allowed to have sex with female rats. Some of the authors suggested that sexual activity in rats increases male hormone level, which produces the larger genital size. Needless to say, because this phenomenon has been demonstrated in rats does not necessarily mean that this phenomenon also takes place in humans. I view the scientific evidence with respect to humans as very inconclusive.

PRACTICAL IMPLICATIONS

There can be no doubt that millions of men would be pleased to have their penises increased in size by the methods described in this chapter. There can also be no doubt that many men who have small penises and are upset by this fact would feel better about themselves if they could obtain an increase in penis size. I wish I could give definitive advice about the effectiveness and safety of these methods. However, I believe that the research evidence is lacking at this time. It does appear that surgery increases penis length, at least in the flaccid state, in some men, and it does appear that surgery increases girth in some men. However, all men do not obtain the expected increase in size, and the penises of some men were better before than after the surgery. All surgery contains risks, and augmentation surgery is definitely not an exception. Furthermore, this surgery is very expensive. If a man is considering augmentation surgery, I would recommend great caution. I would recommend obtaining consultation from at least 3 cosmetic surgeons who do this sort of work and who are not affiliated with each other. I would write down all the questions you intend to ask before the appointment, and I would not hesitate to question the doctor at length. If he is annoyed with the questioning, I would be suspicious. I would check his credentials and reputation in the community with the local medical society. I would also talk with your family doctor. If you have a history of serious mental or emotional illness, it would be well to talk with your psychiatrist or clinical psychologist about your reasons for wanting the surgery.

It is unlikely that penis enlargement would transform an extremely depressed man into an extremely happy man.

I would recommend talking with as many men as possible who have had this surgery, although I must confess that I don't know how you can find them. It is possible that some patients who have had the surgery have given permission to their surgeons to release their names. One limitation of this sort of recommendation is that you may be more likely to talk with the doctor's satisfied customers than his dissatisfied customers.

Vacuum pumps are much cheaper than surgery. They probably involve fewer risks but are probably not risk free. As is the situation with surgery, well-controlled research has apparently not been reported in the medical literature. If one is considering a vacuum pump, I would recommend consulting with your family doctor. I would also talk with several sellers and manufacturers of these devices, but bear in mind that they are in business to make money. A more objective appraisal can probably be obtained from men who have actually used these pumps, or from persons who have at least known of men who have used these pumps. It is possible that urologists in your area have patients who have used vacuum pumps with success, or patients who have used vacuum pumps with no effects, or patients who they have treated for injuries resulting from these instruments.

CHAPTER 9

CONCLUSIONS

My first generalization is that penis size can be important, probably more important than most experts on sexual behavior maintain.

The majority of men would like to have a larger penis. A substantial percentage of women do have preferences with respect to penis size. Some women prefer large, some small, and some medium sized penises. Women who prefer larger penises tend to say that they provide greater stimulation. Women who prefer small penises tend to say that large penises hurt them. Most women don't like penises of either size extreme. It is not known to what extent these preferences are based more on the anatomy and physiology of sexual intercourse and to what extent they are based on psychological factors.

Although penis size is important to many people, as a clinical psychologist I would say that extreme preoccupation with penis size to the exclusion of other aspects of life and interpersonal relationships can be abnormal. If a man spends 10 hours a day attempting to increase the size of his penis, one may question his normality. If a woman spends 10 hours a day searching for a man with a huge penis, one would question her normality. Penis size is not the only important aspect of sex. And, sex is not the only important aspect of life. Having a huge penis is not going to do a man much good when he is 90 years old and dying of cancer. I suspect that family, friendships, religion, accomplishments, and reflection upon a life well spent would provide him with more sustenance than his genital endowment. On the other hand, to deny that penis size is important to many people is a foolish and unrealistic perspective.

Second, although people talk and read more about penis length, for most women penis girth may be more important than length, with respect to sexual pleasure.

Third, most American men probably have a flaccid penis of 3" to 4" inches in length and an erect penis of about 5 1/2" in length. Average diameter seems to be slightly larger than 1" when flaccid and slightly smaller than 1 1/2" while erect.

In proportion to body weight, the infant may have the largest penis of any age group. The penis grows very little from infancy to pre-adolescence. The 11-year-old boy may have the smallest penis in relationship to body size. Most penile growth occurs during early adolescence.

African-American men tend to have larger penises than white men. The difference, however, is greater in the flaccid than the erect state, and greater in length than circumference.

120

Asian-American men tend to have smaller penises than white men.

Methods of increasing penis size include vacuum pumps, stretching apparatus, manual manipulation, and surgery. Solid scientific evidence regarding the efficacy, comparative efficacy, and safety of these methods has not been established.

People for centuries have been fascinated by exceptionally large penises. This has been evidenced in art in diverse cultures. The man with the exceptionally large penis is admired and envied. There are women who fantasize about but not actually want to have sex with a man with a huge penis. Sometimes the penis fantasized is so extremely large that it could not fit into the woman's vagina in real life. Although many people merely want to look at exceptionally large penises, there are people who want such in their sexual activities. This is evidenced by advertisements by women and swinging couples on the Internet and in sexually oriented magazines and newspapers. Men are willing to pay a large amount of money and take the medical risks involved in surgery that purports to increase penis size. The desire of men to have a huge penis is not entirely rational because most women do not crave a huge penis and may find a huge penis painful. Nevertheless, what is entirely rational and what is a feature of the human psyche are two different things. The fascination with the exceptionally large penis cannot be denied, and it may be a fascination of more members of the gender that posses-ses the penis than those of the gender that is ordinarily the recipient of the penis.

Women should be believed when they say that they have genital size preferences and when they talk about pain or discomfort associated with less than ideal genital size compatibility. These women should not be automatically regarded as neurotic, in need of psychotherapy, in need of relationship counseling, or out of contact with reality. Women who prefer a very large penis should not be viewed as animalistic, overly sexed, lustful, or shameful. For some women who prefer longer or shorter penises the situation can be improved by using sexual positions in which there is either greater or lesser penetration. These positions are described in Chapter 7. For women whose partners have too much girth for comfortable penetration and/or sustained intercourse, a lubricant and special partner patience and gentleness should be used. The vagina expands with sexual arousal, and penetration should not take place before this expansion has occurred when such girth incompatibility problems exist. Men with a penis that is "too long" should avoid "poking" movements into the deeper structures of the vagina. Before the assumption of "too long" is made with confidence a women should check with a physician to rule out a number of medical problems that could aggravate the situation or even be the total cause of apparent incompatibility. Penis size should ordinarily not be a major factor in choosing a husband (or in choosing a wife). It may be, however, one factor to consider if one has strong preferences in this regard or if one feels that accommodation to one's own atypical genital size is needed.

One's religious beliefs and commitments to the other person should be considered when decisions are made. Divorce should be one of the last alternatives considered. Sexual abstinence is also a possibility that should seldom be considered by a married couple, but in rare instances it may be an acceptable decision. In spite of the importance of sex stressed by the media, many chaste persons remain psychologically and physically healthy for years.

There may be times when one would want to do nothing and say nothing. Not many men want to hear that their penis is too small for their wife or lover. If a woman receives sexual pleasure and orgasms and satisfaction, there may no good reason to tell a man she wishes his penis were larger. Only a small percentage of women have the lovely face of a beauty contestant. Only a small percentage of men have the handsome face of the great lovers in the movies or the magnificent body of a physique contestant. People are imperfect in many ways, and the world is imperfect in many ways. Perfect genital compatibility is not always possible. And, perfect genital compatibility is not always permanent. A woman may regard a man's penis as too large when she relinquishes her virginity, of perfect size later in her relationship with the same man, and too small after she has borne children and her vagina is larger and less elastic. The purpose of this book is not to make couples obsessed with complete genital size compatibility but to emphasize that many people do have genital size preferences, and that these preferences should be listened to and believed rather than scoffed at. Objective evidence indicates that penis size is important for many people!

WORKS CITED

Adelson, J. P., and W. C. Talmadge. "Tips for Clients: How to Screw Up Your Marriage Counseling." *Family Therapy* 3(1976): 93-5.

Ajmani, M. L., S. P. Jain, and S. K. Saxena. "Anthropometric Study of Male External Genitalia of 320 Healthy Nigerian Adults." *Anthropologischer Anzeiger* 43 (1985): 179-86.

Allen, G., and C. G. Martin. *Intimacy: Sensitivity, Sex, and the Art of Love.* Spokane: Cowles. 1971.

Ard, B. "Penis Size: How Important?" *Sexology* 37 (1970): 19-21.

Arnold, C. B. "Causes of Condom Failure." *Medical Aspects of Human Sexuality* 8 (1974): 8, 163.

Arthaud, J. B. "Silicone-Induced Penile Sclerosing Lipogranuloma." *Journal of Urology* 110 (1973): 210.

Donald I. Templer, Ph.D.

Bahr, R. *The Virility Factor*. New York: G. P. Putnam's Sons. 1976.

Barbach, L. *For Each Other: Sharing Sexual Intimacy*. New York: Signet. 1982.

Blanchard, K., and H. Levine. "Sex and Size: How Men and Women Measure Up Down There." *Marie Claire* (1996, August): 46-50.

Blum, I., R. Marilus, E. Barasch, M. Sztern, S. Bruhis, and H. Kaufman. "Severe Impairment Produced by Morbid Obesity: Report of a Case." *International Journal of Obesity* 12(1986): 185-89.

Burchall, R. C. "What Can Be Done To Increase Sensation in Cases of Vaginal Stretching?" *Medical Aspects of Human Sexuality* 8(1974): 32-47.

Calderwood, D. D. "Male Preference for Anal Intercourse With Female Partners." *Medical Aspects of Human Sexuality* 21(1987): 16.

Chaurasia, B. D., and T. B. Singh. "Anthropological Data of Male External Genitals in Central Indian Healthy Adults." *Anthropologischer Anzeiger* 34(1974): 210-15.

Choi, H. K., I. R. Cho, and Z. C. Xin. "Ten Years of Experience With Various Penile Prosthesis in Korean." *Unsei Medical Journal* 35(1994): 209-17.

Christ, J. E., and J. B. Askew, Jr. "Silicone Granuloma of the Penis." *Plastic and Reconstructive Surgery* 69(1982): 337-39.

Clopper, R. R., J. M. Adelson, and J. Money. "Postpubertal Psychosexual Function in Male Hypopituitarism Without Hypogonadotropinism After Growth Hormone Therapy." *Journal of Sex Research* 12(1976): 14-32.

Cookson, M. S., and P. W. Nadig. "Long-Term Results With Vacuum Constriction Device." *Journal of Urology* 149(1993): 290-94.

Crenshaw, T. L. "How Do Women Feel About Penis Size?" *Medical Aspects of Human Sexuality* 18(1984): 195.

Cronau, H., and R. T. Brown. "Growth and Development: Physical, Mental, and Social Aspects." *Adolescent Medicine* 25(1998): 23-47.

Damon, V., P. Berlier, B. Durozier, and R. Francois. "Length and Circumference of the Penis From Birth to 18 Years and in Relation With the Testicular Volume." *Pediatrie* 45(1990): 519-22.

Danoff, D. S. *Superpotency: How to Get It, Use It, and Maintain It for a Lifetime*. New York: Warner Books. 1993.

da Ros, C., C. Teloken, P. Sogari, M. Barcelos, F. Silva, C. Souto, and P. Alegre. "Caucasian Penis: What Is the Normal Size?" *Journal of Urology* Part 2(1994): 151.

Datta, N. S., and F. B. Kern. "Silicone Granuloma of the Penis." *Journal of Urology* 109(1973): 840.

de Graaf, R., I. Vanwesenbeeck, G. van Zessen, C. J. Straver, and J. H. Visser. "The Effectiveness of Condom Use in Heterosexual Prostitution in The Netherlands." *AIDS* 7(1993): 265-69.

Dickinson, R. L. *Human Sex Anatomy*. Baltimore: The Williams & Wilkins Company. 1949.

Engel, B. *Raising Your Sexual Self-Esteem*. New York: Fawcett Columbine. 1995.

Farkas, L. G. "Basic Morphological Data of External Genitals in 177 Healthy Central European Men." *American Journal of Physical Anthropology* 34(1971: 325-28.

Fisher, R. "Penis Length and Body Height." *Medical Aspects of Human Sexuality* 67(1964): 103.

Flatau, E., Z. Josefsberg, S. H. Reisner, O. Bialik, and Z. Laron. "Penile Size in the Newborn." *Journal of Pediatrics* 87(1975): 663-64.

Friday, N. *My Secret Garden*. New York: Pocket Books. 1987.

Friday, N. *Women on Top*. New York: Simon & Schuster. 1991.

Gagnon, J. *Human Sexuality in Today's World*. Glenview: Scott Foresman and Company. 1977.

Gebhard, P. H., and A. B. Johnson. *The Kinsey Data: Marginal Tabulations of the 1938-1963 Interviews Conducted by the Institute for Sex Research*. Philadelphia: W. B. Saunders Company. 1979.

Getzoff, P. "Penile Shrinkage of Impotent Man." *Medical Aspects of Human Sexuality* 7(1972): 9-80.

Gilbaugh, J. H. *Men's Private Parts*. New York: Crown Trade Paperbacks. 1993.

Goldenson, R. M., and K. N. Anderson. *The Language of Sex From A to Z*. New York: World Almanac. 1986.

Grady, W. R., and K. Tanfer. "Condom Breakage and Slippage Among Men in the United States. *Family Planning Perspectives* 26(1994): 107-12.

Green, R. *Human Sexuality: A Health Practitioner's Text*. Baltimore: The Williams & Wilkins Company. 1975.,

Hawton, K. *Sex Therapy: A Practical Guide*. New York: Oxford University Press. 1985.

Donald I. Templer, Ph.D.

Hite, S. *The Hite Report: A Nationwide Study of Female Sexuality*. New York: Dell Books. 1976.

Jamison, P. L., and P. H. Gebhard. "Penis Size Increase Between Flaccid and Erect States: An Analysis of the Kinsey Data." *The Journal of Sex Research* 24(1988): 177-83.

Jones, K. L., L. W. Shainberg, and C. O. Byer. *Dimensions of Human Sexuality*. Dubuque, IA: William C. Brown Publishers. 1985.

Katchadourian, H. A., and D. T. Lunde. *Biological Aspects of Human Sexuality*. 2nd ed. New York: Holt, Rinehart and Winston. 1986.

Katchadourian, H. A., D. T. Lunde, and R. J. Trotter. *Human Sexuality*. New York: Holt, Rinehart, and Winston. 1979.

Keller, D. E. "Women's Attitude Regarding Penis Size." *Medical Aspects of Human Sexuality* 10(1976): 178-79.

Kinsey, A. C., W. B. Pomeroy, and C. E. Martin. *Sexual Behavior of the Human Male*. Philadelphia: W. B. Saunders. 1948.

Lanson, L. *From Woman to Woman*. New York: Alfred A. Knopf. 1975.

Lighternan, I. "Silicone Granuloma of the Penis: Case Reports." *Plastic and Reconstructive Surgery* 57(1976): 517.

Loeb, H. "Harnröhrencapacitat und Tripperspritzen. *München. med. Wchnschr* 46 (1899): 1016.

Lombardo, J. A., C. Longcope, and R. O. Voy. "Recognizing Anabolic Steroid Abuse." *Patient Care* (1985, August): 2847.

Maltz, W., and S. Boss. *In the Garden of Desire: The Intimate World of Women's Sexual Fantasies*. New York: Broadway Books. 1991.

Masters, W. H., and V. E. Johnson. *Human Sexual Response*. Boston: Little, Brown and Company. 1966.

McCarthy, B. *What You Still Don't Know About Male Sexuality*. New York: Thomas Y. Crowell Company. 1977.

McCary, J. M. *Human Sexuality*. New York: D. Van Nostrand Company. 1979.

Meeks, L. B., and P. Heit. *Human Sexuality: Making Responsible Decisions*. Philadelphia: Saunders College Publishing. 1984.

Money, J., G. K. Lehne, and B. F. Norman. "Psychology of Syndromes: IQ and Micropenis." *American Journal of Diseases of Children* 137(1983): 1083-86.

Money, J., G. K. Lehne, and F. Pierre-Jerome. "Micropenis: Gender, Heterosexual Coping Strategy, and Behavioral Health in Nine Pediatric Cases Followed to Adulthood." *Comprehensive Psychiatry* 26(1985): 29-42.

Murtaugh, J. "The 'Small' Penis Syndrome." *Australian Family Physician* 18(1989): 218-20.

Nakamura, R. "Normal Growth and Maturation in the Male Genitalia of the Japanese." *Nippon Hinuokigakkai Zassi* 52(1961): 72-188.

Nedoma, K., and K. Freund. "Somatosexualni nalezy u homosexualnich muzu. *Ceskoslovenska Psychiatrie* 2(1961): 100-03.

Ortiz, E. T. *Your Complete Guide to Sexual Health.* Englewood Cliffs, New Jersey: Prentice-Hall. 1989.

Pai, G. S., D. Valle, G. Thomas, and K. Rosenbaum. "Cluster of trisomy 13 Live Births." *Lancet* 1(1978): 613.

Phillip, M., C. De Boer, D. Pilpel, M. Karplus, and S. Sofer. "Clitoral and Penile Sizes of Full Term Newborns in Two Different Ethnic Groups." *J Pediatr Endocrinol Metab* 9(1996): 175-79.

Policy Statement of American Urological Association. *Penile Augmentation Surgery*. 1994, January.

Pueschel, S. M., J. M. Orson, J. M. Boylan, and J. C. Pezzullo. "Adolescent Development in Males With Down Syndrome." *American Journal of Diseases of Children* 139)1985): 236-38.

Rabach, J. "Penis Size: An Important New Study." *Sexology* (1970, June): 16-18.

Reed, H. M. "Augmentation Phalloplasty With Girth Enhancement Employing Autologous Fat Transplantation: A Preliminary Report." *The American Journal of Cosmetic Surgery* 11(1994): 85-90.

Renshaw, D. *Seven Weeks to Better* Sex. New York: Random House. 1995.

Reuben, D. *Everything You Always Wanted to Know About Sex*. Toronto: Bantam Books. 1971.

Roen, P. R. "Penile Dimensions." *Medical Aspects of Human Sexuality* 9(1975): 47.

Rosenbaum, M. B. "Sexuality and the Physically Disabled: The role of the Professional." *Bulletin of the New York Academy of Medicine* 54(1978): 501-09.

Donald I. Templer, Ph.D.

Rosenbaum, M. T. "Women's Attitude Regarding Penis Size." *Medical Aspects of Human Sexuality* 10(1976): 174-78.

Rowan, R. L. "Irrelevance of Penis Size." *Medical Aspects of Human Sexuality* 16(1982): 153-56.

Rushton, J. P. "Life-History Comparisons Between Orientals and Whites at a Canadian University." *Person. individ. Diff.* 13(1992): 439-42.

Rushton, J. P. "Asian Achievement, Brain Size, and Evolution: Comment on A. H. Yee." *Educational Psychology Review* 7(1995): 373-80.

Rushton, J. P. *Race, Evolution, and Behavior: A Life History Perspective*. New Brunswick, NJ: Transaction Publishers. 1995.

Rushton, J. P., and A. F. Bogaert. "Race Differences in Sexual Behavior: Testing an Evolutionary Hypothesis." *Journal of Research in Personality* 21(1987): 529-51.

Santini, R. *The Secret Fire: A New View of Woman and Passion*. New York: The Playboy Press Book. 1976.

Schonfeld, W. A., and G. W. Beebe. "Normal Growth and Variation in the Male Genitalia From Birth to Maturity." *Journal of Urology* 48(1942): 759-77.

Shanor, K. *A Study of the Sexual Fantasies of Contemporary Women: The Fantasy Files*. New York: Dial Press. 1977.

Shearer, M. L., and M. R. Shearer. *Rapping About Sex*. New York: Harper & Row. 1972.

Short, R. V. *One Medicine*. Ed. O. A. Ryder and M. L. Byrd. Berlin: Springer. 1984.

Siminoski, K., and J. Bain. "The Relationship Among Height, Penile Length, and Foot Size. *Annals of Sex Research* 6(1993): 231-35.

Smith, A. M. A., D. Jolley, J. Hocking, K. Benton, and J. Gerofi. "Does Penis Size Influence Condom Slippage and Breakage?" *International Journal of STD & AIDS* 9(1998): 444-47.

Stone, H. M., and A. Stone. *A Marriage Manual: A Practical Guidebook to Sex and Marriage*. New York: Simon and Schuster. 1952.

Stuart, S. *The Sensuous Man*. New York: Lyle Stuart, Inc. 1971.

Taguchi, Y. *Private Parts: A Doctor's Guide to the Male Anatomy*. New York: Doubleday. 1989.

Tanner, J. M. *Growth at Adolescence*. 2nd ed. Oxford, UK: Blackwell Scientific. 1962.

Tanner, J. M. *Endocrine and Genetic Diseases of Childhood and Adolescence*. 2nd ed. Ed. L. I. Gardner. Philadelphia: W. B. Saunders. 14-64.

Van De Velde, Th. H. *Ideal Marriage: Its Physiology and Technique*. New York: Random House. 1957.

van Seters, A. P., and A. K. Slob. "Mutually Gratifying Heterosexual Relationship With Micropenis of Husband." *Journal of Sex and Marital Therapy* 14(1988): 98-107.

Wessels, H., T. F. Lue, and J. W. McAninch. "Complications of Penile Lengthening and Augmentation Seen at 1 Referral Center." *The Journal of Urology* 155(1996): 1617-20.

Westney, O. E., R. R. Jenkins, J. D. Butts, and I. Williams. "Sexual Development and Behavior in Black Preadolescents." *Adolescence* 19(1985): 557-68.

Wilkins, L. R., R. M. Blizzard, and C. Migeon. *The Diagnosis and Treatment of Endocrine Disorders in Childhood and Adolescence*. Springfield, IL: Charles C. Thomas.

Zilbergeld, B. *The New Male Sexuality*. New York: Bantam Books. 1992.